How I Got Amazon to Pay Me to Lose Weight and Get in Shape

Working for Bid Bad Amazon

Can be a Real Hoot

ISBN: 9798716345133

Catalog-in-Publication Data is on file
with the Library of Congress

Printed in the United States of America

How I Got Amazon to Pay Me to Lose Weight

Table of Contents

Chapter 1

The Amazon Fitness Club

"Shallow men believe in luck or in
circumstance.
Strong men believe in cause and
effect."
— Ralph Waldo Emerson

To get started, I want you to understand that Amazon does not know I'm writing this book while working as a laborer in the largest Amazon warehouse in Portland, Oregon. Neither have they paid me for writing this book, nor have they had any influence over the story I'm about to relate. While others who have written about working in an Amazon warehouse were doing so under the guise of being "undercover," such was not my scenario. I had no hidden agenda.

When I took the job at Amazon, I really didn't fully know what to expect. I knew from what I had heard and read that I was embarking on a somewhat tough journey. This was due to the company's reputation for almost totalitarian rule over its workforce and demanding working conditions. My situation and reasons for seeking this gig, which I'll fully detail in the next chapter, had nothing to do with turning my escapade into a book. That thought came several months later.

Actually, as the idea of writing about my experiences working at the Amazon warehouse began to germinate in my head, the reason for telling my story became twofold. First of course was the weight loss and physical conditioning, my number one priority. A second reason popped up as I was doing research on what it's like to work at an Amazon warehouse. More on that in a bit.

Here's one general statement I can make with confidence. Complaints about the Amazon workplace being extremely stressful have been overstated by disgruntled ex-employees, over-zealous journalists and crooked political figures. In my experience, most of the stress felt by workers is self-induced. I'll dig deeper into that later, but for now, please trust me that the above statement is true.

A Caveat and My Apologies

There is one important thing I'd like you to understand while you're reading my story. During the first year I worked in the Amazon Warehouse, I saw some amazing business growth – huge increase in volume and ever-growing use of new technology. Hand-in-hand with this growth was the almost constant changes in processes and procedures in warehouse operations. The key takeaway here is that whatever you read about working conditions in Amazon warehouses – whether it be in this book itself or from news articles and media reports on the subject – are time-sensitive. A comment about a certain condition at one point in time may not be valid at a later point due to the constant changes being made.

In addition to the time factor, comments are also facility-sensitive. Not all Amazon warehouses are created equal, and even if that were so, they don't remain identical for long. This is due to the fact that change and improvement initiatives are done at different times from warehouse to warehouse. Change is continuous.

While I'm on the subject of differences, there's a terminology difference I want to introduce. In Amazon parlance, the company has replaced the term warehouse with "fulfillment center" or FC for short. Those two terms are used interchangeably in this book as well as in media communications.

Now, if you're looking for a 'rags to riches' story, please return this book for a refund immediately. One does not get wealthy working at an FC and probably not by writing about it. If you're in line with those thoughts, welcome aboard and enjoy the ride.

So, if you find yourself at one of life's many crossroads, you will probably find my story gives you some valuable food for thought. Regardless of whether or not you find the path I chose at this juncture of my life is applicable to you, the spirit of my reaction to perplexing circumstances will hopefully spark some urge to take action toward whatever goal seems right for you. If you find even one nugget of inspiration from my story, I will find the writing of this book to have been a huge success.

In these turbulent times of a worldwide pandemic, political turmoil and economic uncertainty, we all know people facing tough situations. Whether or not you find this book beneficial to you personally, I'm certain you have friends, family or acquaintances who might get a motivational boost from hearing my story.

A Brief History Lesson

For those of you who don't know the real origin of the Amazon saga or have forgotten what it looked like in the early days, let me fill you in. Amazon was founded by Jeff Bezos in Bellevue, Washington in 1994. It began merely as an online marketplace for books with some rather aggressive blue-sky ideas for explosive growth. I for one was quite skeptical about the odds of this online bookstore ever becoming anything of significance in the retail industry. My basis for this thinking laid primarily in the cost and time delay inherent to the shipping of goods to consumers. How will an online retailer ever compete with the instant gratification offered by shopping malls, not to mention the cost of shipping and handling?

In 1994, Jeff Bezos, a former Wall Street hedge fund executive, decided to jump onto the e-commerce bandwagon with his brainstorm idea for building an online consumer goods marketplace. Investing a modest $10,000 of his own money, he launched Amazon.com as an online bookseller. In the first days of the brash new startup, Bezos and his first few employees packed books and took them to the post office themselves.

He and the small staff spent their time working in his garage on desks made out of doors purchased from Home Depot. Company meetings were held at Barnes & Noble. From the very start, Bezos' stance painted Amazon.com as a technology company whose business was simplifying online buying for consumers and eventually online selling for small and medium size businesses.

Within a few months of the launch, Amazon's annual sales rose to about $1 million. That number continued to climb to nearly $16 million in 1996, and then to $148 million in 1997 and $610 million in 1998. By 2019, company sales hit over $280 billion. Sales were one thing but profitability was quite a different story. The company racked up phenomenal losses year after year for its first 6-7 years of existence. Steadfastly undeterred, Bezos kept funneling all income back into the company to fund growth. I remember shaking my head at the time and thinking to myself, "this can't last much longer." I did not feel Amazon had the staying power, but I was proven dead wrong.

In mid-1997, Amazon went public at $18 per share, giving it a valuation of $300 million. In its initial filing, the company warned investors it expected to continue its "substantial operating losses for the foreseeable future." That did not stop investors and the stock continued its meteoric rise, with only a short respite in 2001 with the dot.com bust. I remember those days rather vividly due to the extensive media coverage. I pondered buying some Amazon stock but decided it was too risky. Financial analysts disparaged the company for its huge investments in technology and marketing while being a mere online book seller.

According to bigcommerce.com, an initial investment of $10,000 at the time of the IPO would today be worth $4.8 million. "Even if you only had $1,000 to invest in 1997, today you'd have more than $626,000." I was just one of the thousands of potential investors who let that one slip by.

Amazon Has Gotten Pummeled

As with many highly successful companies, Amazon has been pummeled with the slings and arrows of detractors from almost every sector of American society. There has been almost nothing written or broadcast in the news media that has been in any way flattering to the company or its billionaire founder. In the spirit of fairness, I thought I should use the book as a vehicle to shine a more positive light on working conditions at Amazon warehouses specifically. That thought turned into the second reason for writing this book.

As an author, I fancy myself as a bit of an accomplished wordsmith. Accordingly, I began to think of words to describe how Amazon has been and continues to be treated in the media and society in general. Terms such as maligned, denigrated, disparaged, and several more came to mind. My list continued to the far end of the negative spectrum to include words like libeled and slandered.

My thought process on this subject had me pondering organizations and prominent individuals I viewed as being treated unfairly by the media and the general public. The list is rather long since it includes people and even entire companies who have gained popularity, or even well-publicized notoriety, due to patterns of unparalleled success in their given field.

Back in the day, IBM was often chastised for its monolithic stature in the computer industry. In sports, the New York Yankees and the New England Patriots garnered vocal enemies based solely on their track records of winning many more championships than other teams. In the modern-day business world, Microsoft got the reputation of being the biggest bully in the high-tech sector. With Microsoft, however, I feel the negative reputation was well-earned by the company's unmitigated greed and monopolistic business practices.

While Bill Gates has been trying to convince the world that he is now a well-intentioned philanthropist and doer of good, his manipulative antics as Microsoft's CEO showed a distinct evil streak to be a key part of his persona.

The crown jewel in my quest for people being treated unfairly had to be found in the political arena, a cesspool of deceit, corruption, character assassination and preposterous lies. Leading up to the 2016 presidential election, I was fascinated by Donald Trump's commitment to "drain the swamp," referring to the terrible conditions the deep state in government had inflicted on American society. While I'm not a big fan of Trump's egotistical personality and oft exaggerated claims, I firmly believe his heart and mind were in the right place as he took drastic steps to improve conditions in the country.

In spite of all the tremendous good Trump did during his 4-year administration, the media, Democrat Party, Big Tech corporations, Google, Facebook, Twitter, supposed educators and many others joined forces to deny him credit for his accomplishments. Instead, Trump was bombarded with vicious accusations of wrongdoing - the ill-advised Mueller investigation, legislative gridlock, election irregularities, phony impeachment proceedings and ramifications of the Covid-19 pandemic.

Here's another sad fact I've observed over the years. People consider it "cool" to criticize and denigrate powerful, competent leaders. Hollywood celebrities who want to appear cool in the eyes of their fan base, were more than happy to join in.

But, let's look at reality. Actors make their living pretending to be someone they're not. They are conditioned to live a lie and the successful ones can make millions doing it. Their huge egos project themselves as being far more important than they are in real life. That air of all-powerful self-importance compels them to step up on stage and pretend to be self-appointed demagogues. Talk show hosts have been getting rich ridiculing every U.S. president for as long as I've been alive. Trump handed them punch lines on a daily basis with his bravado and sarcasm.

In my opinion – and this is based on many years of observing powerful people get denigrated – the vitriol hurled at public figures is more a case of jealousy than anything else. When an average person attacks a person higher up the food chain, they are usually doing it more as a method of elevating their own stature rather than tearing down the accused.

In fairness to all of you who dislike Donald Trump for his egotistical personality and often caustic remarks, I must admit I'm sympathetic toward your feeling. However, I can look past those foibles and see the big picture.

Amazon and Bezos took a severe beating in the press. Unlike Trump's case, Bezos did not light the fire under his detractors with fiery rhetoric. But, it happened anyway.

The Amazon Diet

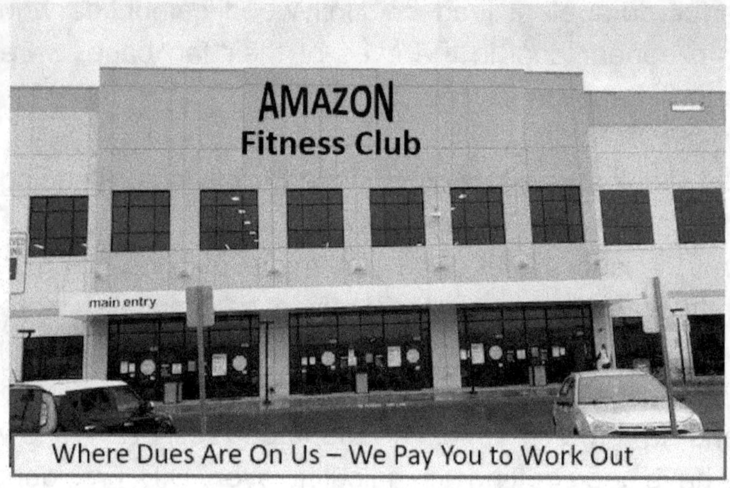

Where Dues Are On Us – We Pay You to Work Out

Stories of people working at Amazon who lose weight due to the demands of the work are plentiful. I encountered many folks who claimed weight reductions of 50, 60, 70 and even close to 100 pounds during their first year. One startling encounter was with a 35-ish female who appeared to be a slim 110 pounds. She smiled when I told her of my 40-pound loss and told me she had lost 80 pounds. 'Babe Alert' flashed through my head. As I began telling co-workers of my weight loss even during my first month on the job, the most common response I got was, "Congratulations, you've discovered the Amazon Diet." I'll get into more details about my own weight loss and improved fitness in the next chapter.

Attitude is everything. The photo-shopped picture above is what I see in my mind when I pull into work each day. Notice that fulfillment center and fitness club both have the initials FC. Coincidence? I think not.

I figured my story of losing weight as a priority reason for seeking work at Amazon would make interesting reading. It did not take long before I found a second reason for writing this book. Finding the working conditions at the Portland Fulfillment Center to be much more tolerable than the accounts I had read, I felt compelled by a sense of fair play to tell the other side of the story. I'll get to that in a minute. Had I put much stock in the media's abject criticism of Amazon, I would probably have steered clear of working there.

As the title of this book portrays, I persevered and succeeded in my quest. By the end of my seventh month on the job, I had lost over 40 pounds and reduced my waistline by six inches. In addition, my previously off-the-chart cholesterol numbers settled back into the healthy range, my pre-diabetes condition was mitigated and the back pain that had plagued me for years became almost unnoticeable. Not wanting to lapse back into my previous condition, I am switching from a fulltime to parttime schedule and will continue working out at the Amazon FC ("fitness club") for the foreseeable future.

While I became enamored with the Amazon Diet, I noticed many of my co-workers either were not interested or incapable of taking advantage of this indirect weight-loss program. It was hard to escape the fact there are a good number of Amazon FC employees who are…well, obese. My first thought when this began to sink in was, "how can so many people avoid losing weight in such a rigorous workplace like this?"

As I climbed the experience ladder, I came to realize many of the worker roles in the FC are not physically taxing at all. Many involve zero amounts of aerobic exercise or muscle exertion. I'll get into those job descriptions in a later chapter.

Sweaty Work Leads to Healthy Outcomes

In retrospect, one of the things I accidentally learned in life is that working hard offers plentiful rewards. Some say that "hard work is its own reward." I'm not sure exactly what that implies but I believe my expanded thoughts on the subject hold water. Speaking somewhat philosophically, I believe that hard work paves the road to a bright future…with the possible exception of doing ten years hard labor in San Quentin.

In my personal experience, working hard equated to higher income on a steadily increasing basis. While in my professional career, hard work did not mean tough physical labor. It had more to do with heavy mental exercise, long hours and persistence. In my younger years, however I did lots of manual labor that was anything but easy. In itself, it was not particularly financially rewarding, but it definitely set a pattern that led to success. The thing that kept me balanced – and in good physical condition – was my "work hard, play hard" focus. My primary recreation involved physical sporting activities.

There is one perplexing contradiction I have noticed over and over again in many peoples' behavior patterns. I've seen many folks go to extremes to avoid working up a sweat at work and then drastically switching gears when they leave the workplace. For many of them, it's off to the gym where they pay dues to work up the same sweat they avoided hours earlier. At the far end of the spectrum are those who pay a personal trainer to make them "feel the burn." Sound familiar?

Working my job at Amazon, several people kidded me about sweating on

> "If you ain't sweatin, you ain't workin'"

the job. I merely chuckled and gave them my standard reply, "well, if you ain't sweatin, you ain't workin'" Some got my point and others went on their merry way shaking their heads as If I was crazy.

From Business Executive to Laborer

Most people who know me feel it's unthinkable that I transitioned from retired business executive to warehouse laborer. You might also think it's quite a bizarre story until you understand all the pieces to this intricate puzzle. In reality, it's proven to be one of the best strategic moves of my life…and believe me, I'm fortunate to say my life has been chocked full of windfalls. My business successes resulted from seemingly drastic changes I've made over the years. I've had lots of adventures, most of them wonderful escapades, faced many interesting challenges and achieved unexpected success. Of course, there have been a few magnificent failures along the way but absorbing lessons learned can be a rewarding experience itself.

In my specific situation, a fairly common set of circumstances pointed me in the direction of an Amazon warehouse for an answer. I'll get into the juicy details in my next chapter, but here's the CliffsNotes version.

I reached retirement age and found myself to be out of shape physically. This was a little distressing since I had always been very active in a variety of sports and other physical activities…at least until the past ten years or so. My jobs in the corporate world largely had me sitting behind a desk except when I was out and about on speaking tours or conducting client workshops.

For the past 5-6 years, I've been ghostwriting and authoring books of my own. That, of course, meant I spent most of my time in front of a computer in my home office, a comfortable but sedentary lifestyle. After completing nine books and getting 75% through a tenth one, I got burned out when it came to writing. I encountered writer's block in a big way. Where once I had enjoyed writing a great deal, now I found it an arduous chore to pound out one more page on the keyboard.

Looking in the bathroom mirror, I realized just how bad things had gotten. My beer belly made it look like I had swallowed a watermelon. How the hell did this happen? Now, I wasn't about to give up hamburgers and beer and I have never had the self-discipline to stick with a diet in my life. Still, I tried again and – you guessed it – I failed once more. Looking down at the dial on my bathroom scale, the depressing number of 210 stared back at me. I know if my scale could talk, it would have yelled, "get off me you fat bastard!"

Over the years, I've always taken pride in my work ethic. I have to credit my father for that. "Hard work is its own reward." I guess that's where I got that thought. At the risk of offending people, I've always felt the 40-hour work week was for wimps. My normal work week has usually been in the 60-hour range. I felt a sort of kinship for Jeff Bezos when I learned he felt the same way. I moved out of my parent's house at age 17 and forged my own path by working hard and then having lots of fun basking in the rewards of my labor. I've been on my own since my teenage years. I was determined to be self-sustaining with no help from my parents or the government. I've never had any regrets because my game plan profited me to the tune of millions of dollars.

But now here I was…in my early 70's and getting fat.

Never having been a stranger to hard work, I vowed to use my well-developed work ethic to end the downward cycle and get back in shape. It was time to get off my butt and get into some serious manual labor. I gave lots of thought to picking the right kind of job to meet my goals. I saw plenty of manual labor types of jobs advertised at the local Amazon warehouse. After doing some research, I decided I'd give it a whirl. What's the worst that can happen?

It's OK to Be Average

Now I'd like to jump to another subject, reasons why many Amazon employees complain about the "miserable" working conditions to misguided news reporters in search of juicy story lines.

It's debilitating to be frequently reminded that your productivity is below average. No argument there. But let's put that aside and look at the big picture. In the grand scheme of life, half of the population is at or below average for whatever is being measured. It's an irrefutable statistical fact. So, if you're labeled as average, don't lose any sleep over it.

I'm not saying people should not be trying to improve because bettering our skill level is a good thing. But consider this – if you're an average worker, it

By definition - 50% of ALL workers are below average on the productivity scale.

simply means half of your co-workers don't do as well as you do. All of a sudden, being average is not the end of the world.

Imagine what would happen to a large company if it would fire the 50% of its workers who fall in the below average category. It's unthinkable and would never happen. So cool your jets and endeavor to stay out of the bottom 10%. As long as employees make the grade as members of this "90% club," Amazon will most likely never fire them for low productivity nor will it affect their wages.

That's probably good news for people who simply want to earn a paycheck and could care less about being a top performer. For the rank-and-file warehouse workers, which is about 90% of the FC workforce by my estimate, there's really no such thing as an annual performance review. I found that somewhat refreshing since I am not a big fan of such annual reviews as I've seen them implemented in most American companies.

I can see the HR folks fuming as they read the previous paragraph. But, let's get real guys. In the majority of cases, annual performance reviews have become little more than wasteful lip service. While HR folks push hard for these reviews, most employees dislike participating in them and most managers dread the yearly process. Having been in management for many decades myself and knowing performance reviews can be quite valuable, I still never looked forward to administering 80% of them.

> **If You Are In the Top 90%, You Have Nothing to Worry About**

It was enjoyable doing them for the top 10% because it was another tool for giving the high achievers the extra recognition they earned. I also enjoyed doing the bottom 10% because I like coaching people to improve. The middle 80% presented the problem. Rather than wait for the annual review cycle to discuss performance with individual employees, I did it as a matter of course throughout the year. So, the annual review was just an exercise in humdrum redundancy in the majority of cases.

Some Guys Are Just Weenies

All other things being equal, one would reason that the physically taxing work many Amazonians are asked to perform would draw more discontent among women than men. We can assume this since males are supposedly the stronger sex. Alas, such is not always the case. Observing my co-workers at Amazon, I came across contradictions to the above assumption. I have heard about twice as many complaints coming from able-bodied men as from women, even though many of the latter weighed in at about 100 pounds soaking wet.

I'll get into some specifics about the physical endurance requirements of certain warehouse jobs when I give you a job-by-job comparison later in the book. But, here I'd like to interject one incident that makes my point. Keep in mind that when anyone – male or female – applies for an Amazon warehouse job, they acknowledge being warned that the job will require them to lift items weighing 50 pounds on a regular basis.

One of the jobs I found to be rather high on the physical exertion scale was that of the down-stacker. This job requires the worker to lift stackable tote containers weighing no more than 30 pounds from a conveyer belt and place them on pallets. Normally, people rotate through this job for periods of 2-4 hours. I've had stints that lasted 8-10 hours and those did drain me.

Another popular "rotating" job is that of the "runner" who uses a pallet jack to move completed pallets to another area of the warehouse. On one long stint of down-stacking, my arms and back were getting tired so I asked one of the runners, a 30ish looking guy, if he would switch with me for the next hour or so. Here was his response. "Hell no, man. Those totes tear my hands up. I can't take it." I commented back, "But these totes all have rounded edges and they have good handles." "Sorry man, I just can't do it," he fired back as he took off with another pallet.

To avoid coming across as someone who thinks Amazon warehouse jobs are like a walk in the park, I do have to admit something. In my early months, I came home almost every day with sore muscles and aching feet – even after I lost the excess weight and got in shape. I purchased a few hand-held massagers, ice packs and a heating pad which I used dutifully after each day's toils. Without them, I probably would not have lasted long.

A not-so-funny incident happened to me on my third day on the job. I was feeling the pain and my back and legs had stiffened up doing my stower job. I went to my boss a little before the lunch break and admitted I might have underestimated how out of shape I actually was. "Unfortunately, I might be ready to throw in the towel," I moaned. "What are my options?

"Well, I have some good news for you," he started. "We know how tough these first few days can be, so we have a practice of asking new employees how they're doing at the lunch break on day three, and that's about right now," he said looking down at his watch. "If employees feel really drained by lunchtime on day three, we let them have the afternoon off – without pay of course." He continued, "…and if they feel they really need it, we allow them to skip work the next day as well."

"Thanks a bunch," I responded immediately. "I will certainly take the afternoon off and hope to be OK tomorrow." As I turned and took my first few steps heading for the front door, my knees wobbled noticeably. "Are you OK? He asked as he grabbed my arm to steady me. "If you want, I can have the guys in first aid bring up a wheelchair to help you get to your car," he offered. "No thanks, I think I'll be OK."

After hobbling down the aisle for about 100 feet, I sat down on a small stack of pallets. Flagging down a guy with a hand-held radio, I explained my situation and my boss' offer of the wheelchair. "I feel like a weenie, but I might like that wheelchair after all."

Needless to say, I felt shamefully helpless as they wheeled me into the first aid office. I was told to lay down on the table and they applied heating pads to my aching muscles. After about 20 minutes, I was able to stand and walk, although still a bit shaky. "Does the offer of taking tomorrow off still stand," I inquired. "Of course it does, and don't feel bad. Your situation is not unusual", they reassured me. "Alright guys, thanks," I said as I headed gingerly toward the parking lot.

How Much Money Do You Expect?

Another complaint I've heard mostly from news reporters and politicians is that Amazon underpays its workers. Sorry, I'm simply not buying that. We've all heard the clamoring from chest-pounding politicians about a $15 minimum wage. Well guess what? Amazon has been paying its warehouse workers $15/hour since 2018.

I'll get into more on that a little later, but my proof point is that I started at a rate of $15.10/hour in 2020 and by the end of my first year, I was pulling in around $40 grand a year – not exactly starvation wages as journalists and politicians would have you believe.

A number of the negative claims about Amazon's deplorable wages and "terrible" working conditions originated in the company's PDX9 warehouse in Portland, Oregon, where I worked. Based on my personal

Snowflake - [sno – flak]
Noun - Someone who thinks they must be treated as special and not subjected to the rigors of traditional society

experiences there, I feel confident in attributing the bulk of negativity to the whining of 'snowflakes' and angry activists intent on stirring up trouble wherever and whenever they can. The snowflake term surfaced in response to the push against the traditional work ethic patterns of the past. At the risk of making too general a characterization, all indications are that the millennial generation prefers a much more relaxed lifestyle.

The new attitude is that the 40-hour workweek is too heavy a price to pay for prosperity and a strong economy. Those should be our birthright they claim. Earning a living should not be such an onerous task. Living off one's parents and spending day after day in their basement playing video games for months on end appears now to be a totally acceptable scenario. In the past, such behavior might have been OK for people in their 20s, but now it's admissible for those in their 30s and often tolerated for 40-year-olds.

Since I predate the snowflakes, I find that while the productivity performance guidelines at PDX9 can be quite rigorous, I found most of them to be within reason from an achievability standpoint. Here's my thought on the subject. If a 70-year old senior citizen such as I can rank in the top 10% of warehouse laborers productivity-wise, why can't people half my age cut the mustard?

Unfortunately, some opportunistic snowflakes think labor unions are probably a good answer to this dilemma.

In February 2021, labor union representatives mustered enough support to force a vote for unionization of the Amazon FC located near Birmingham, Alabama. As this book is being finalized and published, the result of that vote is still uncertain. A similar unionization attempt failed at a Delaware facility in 2014. It is the concerted opinion of me and many of my co-workers at PDX9 that such a move is flat out wrong and will actually harm most workers in the long run.

In today's world, labor unions are obsolete dinosaurs in most cases. While there may be a place for them in a few isolated cases, they have pretty much outlived their purpose. Many decades ago, labor unions were a boon to the working class due to the tremendous power and unscrupulous ways of the elite robber barons and greedy industrialists.

During the past several decades, government laws and regulations have by and large rendered the labor unions redundant. Workers are now well-protected from most of the wrongdoings of industry behemoths. Union leaders however, still yearn for their 6-figure incomes for which they expend no effort other than to agitate the workers against the firms that are giving them wages and benefits. Sorry Bernie Sanders, you're an old, cranky dinosaur who has outlived his usefulness.

The Purloined Pandemic

While I devote an entire chapter later in the book discussing how Amazon handled the 2020 China Virus Pandemic, I'll preview my thoughts right up front in this chapter.

For over a year, we have sat by listening to crooked politicians and misguided journalists run smear campaigns against Amazon and Jeff Bezos for supposed greed and callousness in the company's handling of the pandemic. I was totally bewildered as I watched these bizarre attacks unfold. Nothing could be further from the truth, but then again, the truth doesn't really matter to Amazon's antagonists.

When the pandemic hit with full force, lockdowns and shelter-in-place edicts were ordered causing our society and economy to be thrown into turmoil. Supply chains ground to a halt. The products and services we had taken for granted became almost totally nonexistent. We were left to fend for ourselves. Who can forget the great toilet paper panic of 2020?

The federal and state governments were of little help even though legislators rushed to approve billions and billions of funding. Taking a very dim view of large government and politicians, I was shocked by the $1.9 trillion pandemic relief bill pushed by Democrats. It's mind-boggling that less than 10% of the almost $2 trillion has anything to do with the pandemic. About 90% of it is disgusting pork barrel hand-outs to incompetent political allies. Finger-pointing quickly became commonplace.

Remember when a colossal screw-up by the CDC (Center for Disease Control) delayed corona virus testing for weeks? And what about the lying idiots at the World Health Organization (WHO) claiming China had nothing to do with unleashing the virus on the world? Those are just two of the organizations rewarded with millions of dollars for their deceit and incompetence.

Even while Amazon was being bombarded by its critics for exploiting the public, the company's ability to deliver goods far and wide was a godsend during shelter-in-place orders. It allowed the quarantined masses to receive essential goods without ever leaving their homes. More on this later

The Bottom Line

No one is forcing anyone to work in Amazon warehouses. Applying for a job and exchanging 40 hours a week or so for a living wage does not give one the right to enjoy a utopian workplace. There are plenty of other warehouse and semi-skilled job opportunities out there and people are free to choose one that suits their needs.

Chapter 2

I Was Fat and Happy…Not

"The heaviness of being successful
was replaced by the lightness of
being a beginner again, less sure
about everything. It freed me to
enter one of the most creative
periods of my life."
– Steve Jobs

It has been said that everything comes to an end. Sad but true. Look no further than the fact that death, an event none of us can escape, will be the end for each and everyone of us. Not wanting to get into a philosophical discussion about the possibility of an afterlife, I'll skip that thought and move on.

To truly understand my good fortune of stumbling into the warehouse job at Amazon at the ripe old age of 73, It will help you if I share my mindset with you. After all, most people question my sanity when I call this "good fortune" in the first place. So, bear with me for the next few pages and you'll get some insights about how my crazy mind works. My wife thought I was a little whacko when I told her about my new job. But, as I started losing weight week after week, her skepticism morphed into unexpected esteem. I must admit, her genuine encouragement kept me going strong on those tough days when I came home with aching muscles. It made my experiment even more worthwhile.

Realizing at an early age that I was not going to get out of this lifetime alive, I decided to make the best of it. I dedicated my life to seeking new adventures and having fun. Part of my fun as a teenager was being a renegade. Unfortunately, that put me in the juvenile delinquent category which caused undue stress to my now departed parents. My disciplinarian father told me if I didn't straighten out, I'd end up selling pencils on a street corner. Talk about old school! To this day, I've never seen anyone peddling #2 writing instruments at any intersections in town.

In his infinite wisdom, my dear old dad had two words of advice to me and my siblings: 1) don't bother going to college, you'll just end up as another empty suit, and 2) don't get into the computer field, it's a passing fad. His first point was a welcomed piece of advice since I never liked school anyway. The second really didn't matter since I figured I was never smart enough to be a computer jock of any consequence.

In response to my dad's admonitions, I quit high school at the wise-ass young age of 17 and ran away from home. Actually, I drove away since my dad had begrudgingly allowed me to purchase an old 1952 Chevy with $75 I had made flipping burgers at McDonald's. I put the corn fields of Wisconsin in my rearview mirror and headed for Southern California to become a surfer. I never looked back. That was the beginning of a life of fun times that would last for decades.

Serendipity Is Not a Strategy, But It Works

Fortunately for me, serendipity was on my side. I ended up working as a ranch hand on a small spread just outside of Oceanside, California. Two guys living on the ranch next door taught me to surf and I found myself back in high school at nearby Fallbrook Union High School while I continued my ranch hand duties. Weekends were ideal for surfing of course.

That experience ended when I graduated from high school – smack dab in the middle of the Vietnam war, excuse me, "conflict." The military draft was still in effect with a lottery system for choosing new inductees and guess what. You got it…I had a losing number in the lottery and was certain to be drafted in short order. For fear of ending up in the Vietnamese rice paddies as an army infantryman, I sought cover in the Navy. Damn, the Navy rejected me due to my police record.

Not to be deterred, I marched into the Air Force recruiting office and took the required AFQT (Air Force Qualification Test). Having an above average IQ, I scored at the top of the heap and the Air Force welcomed me with open arms. With my high test scores, the Air Force gave me my choice of career fields. I chose the administrative field where the odds of ending up in the dreaded rice paddies were as close to zero as one can get. So, off to tech school where I could learn to be an admin specialist.

I set the record for the highest graduating score ever for that tech school so the Air Force gave me my choice of base assignments. The school had sort of a "Top Gun" trophy plaque on the wall and my name was at the top. How cool was that? For my base assignment, I chose Oxnard Air Force Base in Southern California - eight miles from the ocean and about 25 miles from Malibu, a famed surfing spot. Naturally I volunteered for night shift duty so I could spend lots of my days surfing.

After about six months on the job, everyone on the base was offered a computer logic test with the top prize being a 3-month computer school gig in Denver and transfer to the base's computer department. Much to my surprise, I took top honors in the school. So much for dad's projection of me selling pencils on the corner. I also learned enough to know that the age of the computer was not a passing fad. Wrong again, dad. Not only that, but I discovered my new passion, an affinity for the computer field. It's important to understand that I had not fallen in love with computers like many computer geeks do, but I truly grasped how computerization could dramatically improve the efficiency and effectiveness of any organization.

After settling into my computer job back at Oxnard, I started looking at what was happening in the computer field in the civilian world. Wow. Starting salaries out in the real world dwarfed the pittance I was receiving from the military. The bad news was that I had over two more years of my four-year stint in the Air Force to serve.

Being an ex-juvenile delinquent, I said to myself, "how hard can it be to get myself ejected from the Air Force?" Being very careful to avoid pushing the envelope to the point where I'd be given a dishonorable discharge or facing some lengthy jail time, I embarked on my strategy to get tossed from the military. After about four months of semi-serious but constant infractions, I had frustrated my superiors to the point of giving me a discharge from the military.

Not only was I free from the stigma of a dishonorable discharge, I even got off without a 'bad conduct discharge' which I admittedly deserved. Instead, I was granted an 'administrative discharge under honorable conditions,' which meant I would still receive the benefits like the G.I. Bill and availability of V.A. home loans.

So, on to the freedom of civilian life and its boundless opportunities. Armed with the fortuitous discovery of my innate computer skills and passion for improving processes with automation, I began a highly successful career in information technology and business management. I enjoyed several decades of six-figure salaries and even one year of seven-figure income. While I had a few stretches that I classified as more work than fun, I have to admit most of my years in the business world fall squarely in the enjoyment category. My career was in line with the famous quote by Mark Twain, "Find a job you enjoy doing, and you will never have to work a day in your life."

Enough past history. Let's get to the more current times. I retired from the IT field about ten years ago by choice. I still wanted to work but had gotten quite bored with the type of work I had been doing. Over the years, I had done a great deal of writing – all non-fiction. I had received lots of praise for my writing from prominent people so I took that as proof I was a pretty talented writer.

I decided my next venture would be that of an author and ghostwriter. Although the books I wrote were well received, none ever hit the best seller list. That's not unusual at all since about 99% of the books ever written never show a profit. Still, I found writing to be a fulfilling endeavor and I earned some nice income for my ghostwriting.

The bad news was that I got so wrapped up in writing, I gradually curtailed the various sports activities I had been doing most of my life. All those physical activities had kept me rather slim and healthy but I lost my motivation for continuing to pursue them. My bad. Sitting at my desk composing documents for a number of years caused my overall wellbeing to gradually deteriorate. I gained weight slowly but surely. My annual physical checkups showed the slippage but I did not pay adequate attention to cause and effect. I simply wrote it off under the category of getting older.

Holy Cow! – How Did I Get This Fat?

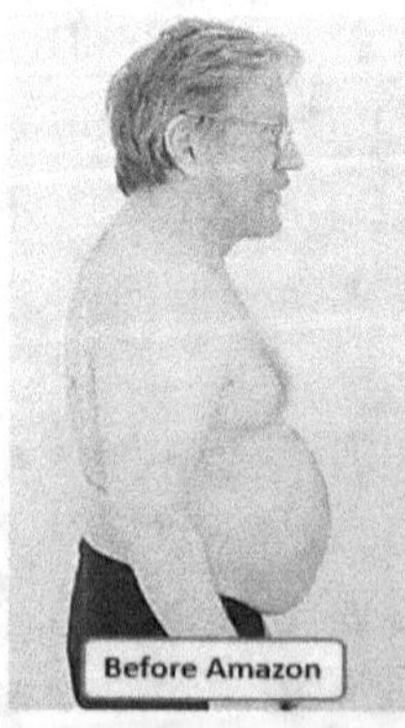

Over the years, I sat by as my weight gradually got out of control. The phrase "sat by" is more than a euphemism here since I literally spent most of my days sitting at my desk. I made mention of this in the previous chapter. As I said, I tipped the scales at a disgusting 210 pounds. If I was 6'2" I guess 210 would be an OK number. But, yikes, I'm a mere 5'7" and that's unacceptable.

Since my old surfing days, I had developed a serious affinity for spending time at the beach. If I wasn't surfing, I was running in the sand. I became quite an adept runner, falling just short of the 4-minute mile at San Diego State. My love for the beach drew me repeatedly to the Caribbean and I've taken about 40 vacations there over the years. Having gained all that weight, I'd be embarrassed to set foot on a beach again. Something had to change.

There were other indicators that raised some red flags as well. My doctor had been bugging me for several years about my above average cholesterol levels and had put me on a regimen of anti-cholesterol meds to get that under control. She did mention the fact that regular exercise would help lower the cholesterol count.

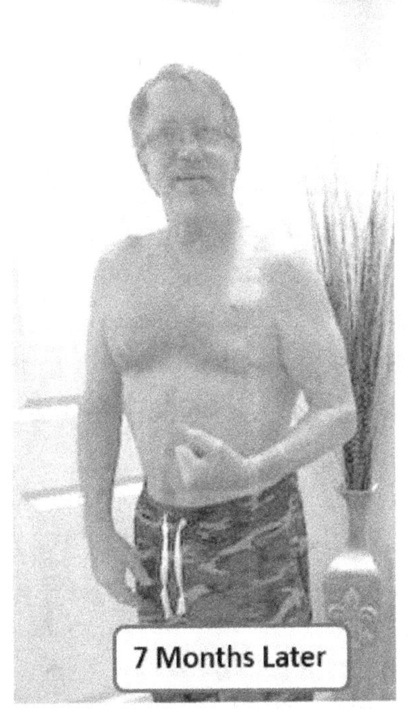
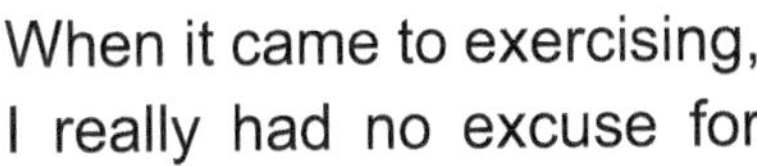

When it came to exercising, I really had no excuse for avoiding it. For years, I had been an accomplished runner but when I developed shin splints 20 years ago, I decided it was time to 'just not do it' any longer – sorry Nike, you're history. While I had curtailed by daily runs, I simply had no valid excuse for not exercising. When I turned 65, I was pleasantly surprised to learn that my Medicare Advantage insurance plan included free membership to a nice selection of health clubs. I had started going to 24 Hour Fitness several times a week but gradually lost interest and that good habit went into the ditch. Even though it was free, I just could not muster up the self-discipline to make workouts at the club a regular practice.

At my last physical, my doctor found signs of a pre-diabetic condition in my annual blood test. Great. Diabetes? What the hell is happening to me? Merely being over 70 years of age should not be a valid excuse for being in poor health.

Bigger Belly = Smaller Life Span

It was now painfully obvious to me that I was at another crossroad in my life and this one had some pretty serious consequences. The choice was obvious, either lose weight or continue to spiral downward into the darkness. The ultimate destination I was headed for was not at all appealing. I've had a fabulous life and I'm not going down without a fight. Call me greedy but I want more fun times.

Looking back over the past several decades, I had always been relatively slim and trim. When I look around at today's younger generation, I see lots of obesity. It's not my imagination. Statistics prove my observation is right on. In spite of all the years I spent in pretty good shape, I still ended up terribly overweight. My bad. But, what does that portend for today's youth. Without a healthy head start, what shape will they be in when they reach retirement age? I shutter to think about it. However, that's a subject for another book, so let's move on.

I know what you're thinking. Why not just go on a diet? I've tried dieting before and realize I'm not cut out for it. The bottom line is that just like the health club dilemma, I simply lack the self-discipline for limiting what I eat and drink. The thought of giving up burgers and beer…well, it's just not in the cards for me.

Since one of my many positions in corporate America had been that of a high-level research analyst, I saw it was in my best interests to get more knowledgeable about the health effects of being overweight.

Here's a summary of what I discovered.

The negative health effects of being overweight or obese occur more in people of middle age or higher. Shedding pounds may prevent, slow, or even reverse many of them. Here's the list I compiled of the downside effects of carrying around too many pounds.

- All-causes of death – an ominous generality
- High blood pressure (Hypertension)
- High cholesterol
- Type 2 diabetes
- Coronary heart disease
- Stroke
- Hardened Arteries leading to poor circulation
- Kidney Disease
- Gallbladder disease, gallstones
- Osteoarthritis
- Breathing trouble
- Worsening asthma and COPD symptoms
- Fatty liver disease, cirrhosis
- Gout - built-up uric acid causes joint pain
- Sleep Apnea

- Increased likelihood of cancer

Source: webmd.com

An 'All In' Sort of Guy

I realized years ago that life without working some sort of job was of no interest to me. Without something meaningful to do regularly, I feel kind of lost. By meaningful, I don't mean it has to involve accomplishing great things. Been there, done that. It simply has to be something involving a purpose, regardless of how underwhelming the mission might be.

I tried retiring from work in my mid-60s with visions of playing lots of golf with my buddies. After several months spent on the fairways and greens trail, I found there are only so many rounds of golf one can play before even that gets somewhat boring.

The obvious solution was to find a job that would force me to exercise. Again, I know what you're thinking. Why not simply work part time? That would be a wise choice, but unfortunately I'm an 'all in' sort of guy. Whenever possible, I always go for the gusto. So I decided to roll up my sleeves, get off my lazy ass and go do some serious physical work. Besides, my writing could wait. In fact, I really needed a break from writing day in and day out anyway. Similar to my corporate career, writing had lost much of its luster and it was time for a new adventure.

Chapter 3

Getting Hired and Getting Fired

"Although no one can go back
and make a brand new start,
anyone can start from now and
make a brand new ending."
- Carl Bard

I hope I didn't bore you by taking the previous chapter to provide you with the background information that led me to seek a job in an Amazon warehouse. I felt it was necessary to set the stage for the rest of the book. I thank you for sticking with it. By understanding my mindset and motivation, you'll have a better reference point as you take in the rest of what I have to say about what it's like to work in an Amazon warehouse. The prism through which I looked as I observed the work environment is substantially different than that of almost every other employee. Being more emotionally detached from the day-to-day drama, I like to think my observations and opinions will give you the most objective viewpoint you'll get on the subject.

So, now that you're armed with all the background information you need, let me begin the saga of my fulfillment center experience.

How does one embark on a job search when you're over 70? On this subject, I have a leg up on most people. Two years ago, I wrote a book called "Gig Economy: The Good, The Bad and the Ugly" for which I did some good research on the job market. While I was not looking for a 'gig,' which in the new economy refers to temporary employment, parttime jobs or independent contractor work, my research certainly equipped me with the knowledge of where to look for all kinds of jobs.

My first stop was Craig's List for the Portland area, which covers Portland and the surrounding geography. Eyeballing the various job categories, I selected the "General Labor" section as the place I figured I could find a job that required little more than physical work. Salary didn't really matter since I have plenty of income with Social Security, a few pensions and my retirement investments. I also didn't need an employee benefits package since Medicare and Medicare Advantage cover everything I need as far as medical expenses go.

Of course, now that Joe Biden has been elected president, the situation with Medicare Advantage will probably change in the next few years. Biden and his Democrat cronies have all promised to eliminate all private health insurance as a key part of the Green New Deal. According to the Democrat Party, the elimination of private health insurance is necessary to make 'Medicare For All' feasible. The logic there escapes me, but then so does the financial feasibility of most of the Green New Deal. I don't know if many people truly understand that Medicare Advantage is not a government program, but in fact private health insurance. So, unless something drastic happens in the political sector, Medicare Advantage will be a thing of the past. Since Medicare itself is realistically insufficient to provide anything more than bare bones health insurance, millions of people may be seeking employment only to get healthcare benefits.

Fairly prominent in the General Labor category were several job listings for warehouse positions with Amazon, which has several warehouses in the Portland area. The largest of these locations is in Troutdale, OR about a 20-mile drive from my house. They had open positions at Troutdale and the ad said to drop by and apply at the warehouse, no appointment necessary. As I recall, the ad specified a $15/hour starting wage, no experience necessary but applicants must be able to lift 50-pound boxes without assistance and to be able to stand for most of the standard 10-hour shift.

I immediately did a Google search to get comments and opinions on what it is like to work in an Amazon warehouse. As I expected, virtually all of the comments I found were negative, some being outright inflammatory. In reality, who is going to post a positive review of a minimum wage type job? I took the reviews with a grain of salt and made the short drive to Amazon's warehouse that afternoon.

Organized Chaos

Upon my arrival at the Troutdale facility, I went to the main entrance and was directed to the hiring office at the far end of the building. The place was huge. As I neared the hiring office, I got my first glimpse of how chaotic the place was. That would sink in more over the course of the next few days. The hiring office was jammed with people. Keep in mind this was in late March of 2020 and the Covid-19 pandemic was still in first gear. In fact, the word pandemic was not even in use at the time. There were stickers on the sidewalks and inside the building warning people to stay six feet apart, but enforcement was pretty lax.

I walked up to a guy wearing an Amazon jacket and an official looking name badge. "Is this where I apply for a job?" I inquired. "Do you have an appointment?" was his curt reply. "Ah, no I don't," I said, "The ad said just to stop by and no appointment is needed." I instinctively knew where the conversation was headed. "Well, we're all booked up for today," he informed me. "Tell you what…give me your name and cell phone number and I'll book you a slot for tomorrow," he offered. "Will there still be openings tomorrow?" He laughed and assured me, "Damn right. We pretty much hire everybody willing and able to work. You'll probably be hired on the spot. What's better for you, morning or afternoon?" "Morning works for me," I replied. He set me up with a 10:00 AM appointment time.

After getting dressed in attire appropriate for working in a warehouse, I showed up at Amazon at a little after 9:30 the following morning. After checking in with the guy at the front door, he directed me to the "10:00 appointment line"

– wow, a separate line just for the 10 AM applicants. I took my place as number 4 in line, standing dutifully six feet behind the #3 lady in keeping with the 6-foot marks on the sidewalk. The line grew to about 25 people in ten minutes. Most of the people I spoke with had just lost their jobs due to the China virus epidemic, as it was being called at the time. I thought: I guess this is what they mean by 'cattle call.'

As 10 AM approached, we were told we could get in line behind the last of the 9:30 folks waiting for their turn to approach the front desk. At the huge front desk were four Amazonians standing in front of computer screens. There was no application to fill out and certainly no need for a resume. All we had to do was sign a form agreeing to submit to a drug test and background check. While I was awaiting my turn in line, I watched several people make a U-turn and head for the exit. I could only assume they were freaked out because of the drug test requirement. I learned later the drug testing had been temporarily suspended due to the large volume of applicants. Sorry folks, you bailed out too soon.

The 'processing in' step consisted of having our photo taken and watching a 10-minute "Welcome to Amazon" video. We were told the normal new employee orientation sessions were no longer being done on-sight due to lack of room for proper social distancing. Instead, we were told we'd have to go home and watch the online orientation video before we could start work.

I guess this meant I was hired but no one told me whether I was or wasn't. "I suppose so," was the response I got from the HR guy who was in charge of showing the video.

"Just go sign on and watch the orientation video and you'll be given a start date," he offered as a way of implying yes. I was given a lanyard for my employee badge but no badge. HR told me I'd receive that the first morning I report for work. I went home, got on the Internet and went to the HR orientation website. I tried to start the orientation session about 20 times over a frustrating 2-hour time period. All I got was a message saying, "Cannot connect." Finally giving up with the Internet approach, I called the HR phone number I was given. After spending a good 30-40 minutes on hold, I was told their orientation website was jampacked due to the sheer volume of new hires. "Keep trying," was about all they would say.

After about 4 hours or so, I was finally allowed into the online orientation session. I had been told the orientation would take 3-4 hours. As I now recall, the on-line session took considerably less than an hour. A few hours after finishing, I received an email from Amazon's HR department saying I should show up for work the next morning at 7:00 AM. Great, I guess I was actually hired.

It was the first thing in the morning of my supposed day one of employment at Amazon that I ran smack dab into my introduction to the company's state of 'organized confusion.' "Sorry Mr. Kuiper," the person in charge told me. "I have no badge for you. Did you complete the orientation and complete all the online forms?" I assured them I had and produced an email saying I had done so and was cleared to start work. The HR person apologized for the mix-up but all she was allowed to say was, "You'll just have to come back tomorrow and hopefully you'll have better luck."

Better luck? What is this, the Amazon employment lottery? In fairness to the HR onboarding folks, I understand that amidst the epidemic chaos, not everything could be expected to run smoothly. So, back home I went.

As I pulled into the parking lot at 6:45 the next morning – now my official day two – I felt fairly confident Amazon would have straightened out the situation during the previous 24 hours. Not so, I realized as I was again told they had no badge for me. "You'd better go to the hiring office on the corner and see what's causing the delay," I was told. "It's probably a form you forgot to fill out." Then it hit me. Amazon's rule number one is this: the company is always right, and the employee is always wrong. Sounds a little harsh on my part, but I later found I was mostly right on this point in general.

The Human Resources Conundrum

I must digress for a minute with an observation that summarizes my view of Human Resources departments in corporate America. Remember back in the day before the "HR" moniker was invented, when this entity was generally known as the payroll department? OK, maybe you're too young, but trust me this is a fact. As recruiting and new employee onboarding became more sophisticated over the years, the old payroll department was renamed "Personnel." At least they acknowledged we were still persons.

Then came the flood of legislation and lawsuits as the employee rights cause embraced the business world. Front line company workers perhaps made a little more money and surely got better employee benefits via the movement. But, hordes of human rights lawyers got rich beating up on businesses for any hint of employment unfairness.

That led to the inception of the term Human Resources and the department of the same name. So, we the people now became "resources" not unlike raw materials and production equipment. At least they acknowledged the human aspect of our beings. The former payroll clerks gradually morphed into "HR professionals" and got hefty pay increases. The department was elevated from its former standing as a component of the comptroller's office to a high-level organization reporting directly to the company's CEO, and occasionally wielding more power than the CEOs themselves. We can thank the government and the lawyers for this. I personally observed this gradual metamorphosis during my 50+ years in the business world.

At the risk of an over-generalization, I'll go out on a limb and say that today's HR departments in American business have an above average number of pompous staffers obsessed with their own importance and power. From their legally protected ivory tower, they look down with disdain on other employees, even company executives. Many careers have been relegated to the compost heap due to a single complaint to HR, even if it was never confirmed in a court of law.

The very term "HR" conjures up fear in the hearts of many business people. Being summoned to HR is the adult equivalent of being sent to the principal's office back in our school days. It's not simply a coincidence that Dilbert creator Scott Adams chose to establish the persona of

Catbert, the evil HR Director in his cartoon parody of the American workplace.

Having said all that, I'll step down off my soapbox and add a very important footnote. There are many honest and well-intentioned people in HR departments trying their best to ensure a fair and equitable workplace for all employees. This segment of HR people has not adopted the "holier than thou" arrogant attitude that has become fairly common in HR organizations. I was pleasantly surprised to encounter many genuinely friendly and helpful people in the PDX9 HR department. In short, they were probably among the most pleasant HR folks I have met over the years.

Easily Hired!, Readily Fired?

Having started this chapter with my account of how swiftly and chaotically new employees are hired at Amazon warehouses, I'll switch to the other end of the spectrum – the odds of and fuzzy uncertainty of being fired. It seemed to me that from day one on the job, warehouse employees are purposely kept on edge about the likelihood of being unceremoniously terminated. I'm sure everyone has heard of the "carrot and stick" management technique where the carrot is a potential reward and the stick is a possible punishment. In my time at the warehouse, I frequently saw both veiled and outright threats of stick use but any mention of carrots…well, the subject rarely came up. In reality, this did not surprise nor disappoint me. I had worked in a few warehouses in my early days and found relatively few "carrots" being used to tempt minimum wage workers to strive for excellence. In fairness to Amazon, the "stick" was the most common motivator across the board.

The 2-word phrase "written up" is the most prominent threat of "stick" usage in the FC. It is meant to strike fear in the hearts of employees who are falling short of expectations, either because of low productivity, mistakes or rule violations. Although I pride myself to be a high productivity, rule-following kind of guy, I must admit the 'getting written up' line came my way on a number of occasions. Since I really don't need to have or keep a job, I was able to avoid letting it bother me. But for the average warehouse worker, I could see it to be a rather effective intimidation tool. I never found out if Amazon managers are taught to use that technique or if they simply pick it up from their peers.

In a 2019 article from *The Verge* entitled "How Amazon automatically tracks and fires warehouse workers for productivity," a reporter commented on the rate of warehouse terminations. The article states, "an attorney representing Amazon said the company fired hundreds of employees at a single facility between August of 2017 and September 2018 for failing to meet productivity quotas. A spokesperson for the company said that, over that time, roughly 300 full-time associates were terminated for inefficiency." Assuming the 300 was close to being accurate - and it appears to be – the reporter claimed, "that would mean Amazon was firing more than 10 percent of its staff annually, solely for productivity reasons."

Now for a dose of reality. The figure of 300 people getting fired in the course of a year initially seems drastic. But, if we step back for a look at the bigger picture, it amounts to only 10% of the worker population. Still too high, you say? Would it shock you to learn that former General Electric

CEO Jack Welsh, one of the most respected business executives in history, used that very figure in his famous argument that "leaders should fire the bottom 10 percent of their workforce each year, as part of an orderly continuous improvement process." My first thought about Welch's rule is that it is not sustainable year after year. In normal settings, I think I'm right on that. But what about situations like Amazon's where the annual turnover rate is 100% or higher? Suddenly, it appears to be a wise move.

During my time at Amazon, I saw that managers have far less control of their workforce than in other companies. Key decisions like hiring, firing and personnel scheduling appear to be made more by automated software programs than by managerial judgment. Notice I did say "appear" so I've left myself a little wiggle room. Before you get sucked up in the "Amazon warehouses are run by computers" rabbit hole, let me dispel that as a myth which obscures the truth at Amazon and other large corporate operations.

What It Takes to Get Canned

Unlike most of the people who work in Amazon warehouses, I didn't need the job because I obviously was not doing it for the money. There was a wide array of jobs which would have given me the physical exercise I wanted to achieve my goals. Almost all of them paid less than Amazon's starting wage, but the hourly rate was not part of my decision-making criteria.

Such was not the case for the majority of my co-workers because the lower wages at non-Amazon jobs was simply not adequate for their financial situations. This gave me a different perspective about working conditions, especially concerning the prospects of being terminated. I was fortunate in that any threats or intimidation involving the loss of my job meant nothing to me. Well, I must admit that's not totally correct. I believe almost no one is immune from the trauma of being fired from a job. It still hurts because it's an indicator of incompetence.

Still, I was quite interested in finding out the real story behind the commonly held belief that Amazon warehouse workers get fired more often than their counterparts in other companies. This was around the same time thoughts of writing a book about my experiences was marinating inside my brain. My research into this subject had to be done in stealth mode since I assumed that it would be grounds for termination.

If anyone in management found out I was writing a book about working conditions in the warehouse, that might have ended my physical fitness plans. I had already found two other books on the subject written by ex-insiders and both were highly critical of everything Amazon. Even though I sensed my book would have far more positive opinions than negative criticism, I would not expect company management to take my word on that.

Much of my early investigative inquiry activities were with low-level employees like me with whom I'd strike up conversations during breaks and lunch periods. With social-distancing practices being enforced, private one-on-one conversations were very difficult to conduct. Adding to that was the fact that the informal grapevine of scuttlebutt was only a fraction of the size of those in other organizations due to Amazon's laser-like focus on minute-by-minute productivity. This left little time for interpersonal chitchat. Not a dig against Amazon, simply the reality of the situation.

One telling fact I uncovered was the small number of people that were with the company for more than six months. That helped confirmed what I had read about the extremely high turnover rate. It also solidified the notion that an active grapevine was all but nonexistent. Very few people I spoke with had any knowledge of other employees being fired or even "written up" for transgressions. Most of the grumbling was about the monotony of the work and I could attest to that myself. But what does one expect from a minimum wage type job. Personally, I had no expectations of anything mentally stimulating, much less cognitively challenging.

Around the time I finished the second month of my employment tenure, an unexpected opportunity popped up. My then current boss asked me if I'd like to take on a 30-day stint in the receiving department. Being bored and somewhat underwhelmed by the stowing gig I had from day one, I jumped at the chance. He stressed the fact that it was only for 30 days, but I was glad for the break. So, on to Receiving I went with a spring in my step. I tried to always keep a positive attitude about the job…well, because that's how I roll. I'd always kept that attitude about work and it had served me very well during my career.

The Receiving Department afforded employees more variety in their day-to-day work activities than did the Stow area. With minimal training, one could rotate through a number of roles in the department, which was adjacent to the receiving dock - usually a hotbed of activity. Unlike stowing, workers in receiving did not work in isolation from each other. While the focus was still on minute-by-minute productivity, it did provide more leeway for cross-talking between co-workers. We did not get the feeling that a manager or his henchmen were always staring over our shoulders monitoring our every motion and watching for missteps in our actions.

It was in Receiving that I was able to form a few relationships with other workers. I actually began to know first names and mold a few loose friendships. It also afforded me the opportunity to speak with more senior people who had been around for more than a few short months. Further, this gave me the input I wanted to get my arms around the employee termination issue. One of the opening lines I'd use that garnered some valuable insights went like this, "Just out of curiosity, what does it REALLY take to get fired here? How concerned should I be that I may lose my job?"

As one would expect from an environment like that of a large Amazon FC where turnover is high and manager training appears somewhat spotty, questioning the status quo does not go over well. The inquiries I made drew a wide variety of responses from one end of the spectrum to the other. The more jaded responders were prone to be a bit harsh with comments like, "You'd better watch your back – they will fire you on the spot if you're not towing the line." On the other hand, I got many non-committal responses like, "Good question, I really don't know. Some people get away with murder and others lose their jobs over minor incidents."

So, by the numbers, exactly why do people get fired? Only HR really knows and they are being tight-lipped on the subject. As one would expect, there are no figures on this published. The gossip grapevine is of little help in this area, not by management directive but by the nature of FC worker isolation. The "heads down, limited chatter" nature of the work environment does not facilitate employee cross-talk. Keep in mind here that my time in the PDX9 FC was during the corona virus pandemic so Amazon's tightly enforced social-distancing was a huge factor in limiting the gossip grapevine. During breaks, people were kept six feet apart and typically separated by mylar cubicle walls.

From my informal survey, here are the common reasons for getting fired, ranked in order of occurrence.
- Below average productivity
- Excessive TOT (Time Off Task)
- Drug use, including failing random drug tests
- Excessive time on mobile phones instead of working
- Exceeding UPT (Unpaid Time) allotment, i.e. missing too much time at work

The "Computer Did It" Cop-out

For most managers, having to fire subordinates is not a pleasant experience. As a former business manager myself, it gave me no sense of enjoyment. In fact, it made me question my own skill set. Where did I fail to give this person what they needed to succeed? One thing I did not do was point the "firing finger" at someone or something else. I took full responsibility for the decision because the buck stopped with me.

When I refer to "something else," I'm speaking primarily of the employee productivity charts managers get on their laptop screens. The image below is my "re-creation" of approximately how those screens look. Since being able to review those screens was above my pay grade, I am only able to create a rough version of how they appear.

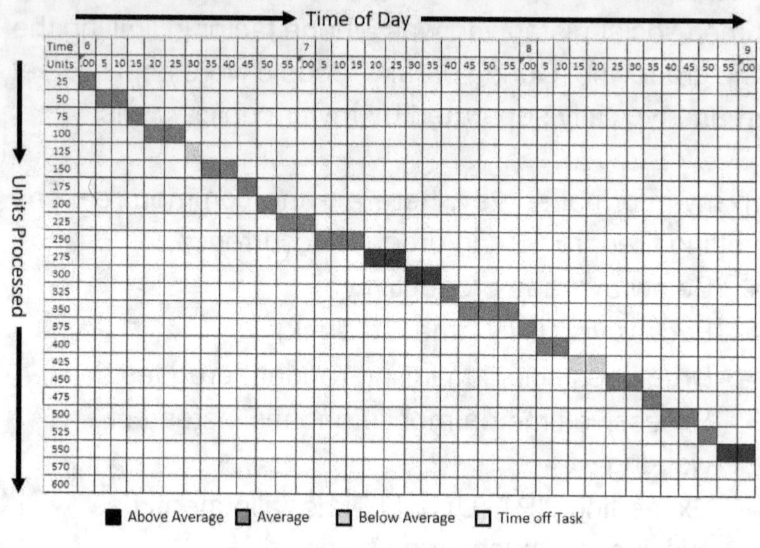

Daily Productivity Analysis

I believe this "buck stops here" mentality may not apply to FC managers. This may not be 100% accurate but I assume there is almost always someone behind the curtain applying pressure to fire those ranking low on the productivity totem pole. I think managers really have to stick their necks out to save a statistically weak employee from the chopping block.

Personally, I cannot truly fault Amazon managers for not always stepping up to the plate to protect employees who appear to fall into the unacceptable category on productivity graphs. Having seen enough about the high level of sophistication built into Amazon's productivity evaluation tools, I can assume the analytics are multi-level. While first level statistics are evaluated at the individual worker level, I would bet big bucks they are summarized upward to the various levels of management responsibility. Computer programs are almost never able to incorporate soft factors like observational judgment into their statistical calculations. And therein lies the rub.

With the exception of Artificial Intelligence (AI), computers cannot and do not think for themselves. They need to be programmed by humans to perform complex analytics to produce the charts, graphs and reports used in decision making. Having been an IT professional myself for many decades, this is certainly not an earth-shattering reveal. Nor is it for most experienced business people. I feel I need to point out this simple fact because a surprisingly large number of people seem to be unaware of this basic truth.

Perhaps it's an overzealous and uninformed media or some opportunistic sci-fi movie producers who have perpetrated this hoax. They have instilled the fear in many otherwise rational people that business computers are poised to take over the world. This is not to say that computerization has not made some jobs obsolete through automation, but the paranoia has gotten out of hand in several areas.

The bottom line is this. Computer programmers are human – perhaps a little anti-social and reclusive in many cases – but human nevertheless. But in almost all cases, computer programmers are not the ones deciding which statistics to evaluate and which actions to be taken as a result of analytical outcomes. Other humans direct programmers concerning what data to collect, how to analyze it and what criteria is used to suggest solutions and/or corrective action.

At Amazon, like other companies, it's the people behind the "curtain" who make the logical - or sometimes illogical - decisions that draw criticism. Many of those human decision-makers, however, often fail to own up to the role they played in the game when things go awry. As I see it, angry ex-employees complain they were fired by a computer and an amateur journalist latches onto the story and paints the company as an evil monster. Then, an unsuspecting public takes the ludicrous charge at face value. Seldom does anyone step forward to set the record straight. It's sometimes more convenient to let inanimate computers take the blame.

I have witnessed both sides of the issue during my tenure at Amazon. I'm paraphrasing here but I've been on the receiving end of reprimands that go something like this, "I don't personally have anything against your performance, but the computer shows you're making more errors than you should. If this continues, I guess I'll have to write you up."

Here's one actual incident that solidifies my point. It occurred while I was working as a stower (one who places incoming goods into inventory bins) in my first month of employment. While working at my station, I was approached by one of my manager's henchmen carrying a laptop and staring at the screen with a disapproving look on his face. "I have a few questions as I'm looking at your performance record," he started.

Pointing to a spot on a graph, he started, "I see that yesterday between 8:13 AM and 8:21 AM, you didn't record any work being done. Can you tell me what you were doing during those eight minutes?" "You've got to be kidding," I thought to myself. Eight minutes? Yesterday morning?

"I have no idea. Can you tell me what YOU were doing at that time?" I fired back sarcastically.

"Don't be a wise ass. I'm just trying to help you improve."

"Sorry, I'm simply trying to point out that almost no one is going to remember what they were doing during a specific eight-minute period of time over 24 hours ago"

"OK, so how about the end of the day? The record shows you logged off your work station at 5:29 PM (end of shift was 5:30), but you didn't clock out of the building until 5:40 PM. Are you telling me it took eleven minutes to walk to the front of the building?"

"I think that's probably right. Yesterday I was working on the third floor at the west end of the building and the time clock is two floors down and a long walk away. Besides, I'm 70 years old, my legs were kind of tired from standing all day and I guess I can't walk as fast as you young kids."

"Well, I'm not going to write you up on this but try to do better."

As he walked away in a huff, I wondered if coming to work at an Amazon was not a very smart move.

I must interject here that not all FC managers and supervisors fall into the 'cold-hearted, by the numbers' category. While working in the Receiving department, I had the pleasure of working for an astute boss who shed some light on the productivity monitoring scenario. A few weeks after he was added to the department staff, he approached me with his laptop open and I could see he was looking at the graph depicting my minute-by-minute productivity performance. I thought to myself, "Oh crap. Here we go again with the 'try to do better' spiel."

Pointing to some numbers on the graph, he started the pitch I had heard before. "Looking at your productivity numbers from yesterday, I see you ranked a little below average in number of units processed per hour. Compared to your numbers from last week, it looks like you slipped a bit. Is there anything you need that will help move these numbers a little higher?"

Since he was obviously open-minded on the productivity ranking scenario, I saw an opening to share my thoughts. It was refreshing to encounter a manager who was asking for input rather than rushing to judgment.

"Well boss," I started. "I'm sure you understand that not all products we handle are created equal." He nodded in agreement so I continued. "I receive everything from single greeting cards to cases of soft drinks. From a numbers standpoint, both a greeting card and a case of pop count as a single unit. I don't have to tell you the difference between receiving a hundred greeting cards and a hundred cases of soft drinks. Often, the mix of products we receive varies dramatically during the course of a day, so the number of units processed per hour averages out over time – but not very quickly in many cases."

"Of course I understand that," was his response.

Realizing the conversation was on the right track, I continued. "Recalling my activities of yesterday, I remember having an almost constant stream of big-ticket items – lots of cases of Red Bull and such, 12 pound jugs of laundry detergent and stuff like that. I got few if any of what I call 'trinkets' which are the small products such as ribbons and bows and bottles of vitamins. Thinking back to last week, I was pleased to be flooded with thousands of trinket type items."

The boss kept nodding so I kept talking.

"Please understand this is not my first rodeo," I continued. "During my corporate career, I spent huge amounts of time in the inventory management arena, even to the point of designing systems that measured the productivity of people processing inventory. One thing I learned was that looking purely at the number of units processed per time period can be misleading, especially in the short term. This very same issue came up when I worked as a stower. With all due respect, I feel that Amazon's heavy focus on monitoring units per hour to rank worker productivity is sometimes a little short-sighted." With that, I rested my case.

My boss' response to my venting was better than I expected. In fact, it was perfect. He assured me that his method of evaluating employee performance went well beyond the statistics on a graph. "I use my personal observations of individuals working on the line as I evaluate worker productivity. I can tell the difference between the hard workers and the slackers just by observing people. Don't worry too much about these graphs. I use them only because we have to as part of our reporting process."

The subject never came up again, which speaks well for PDX9 management. While there are a few "hard ass" managers skulking around, I found those who were generally concerned about their workers to be in the majority.

Chapter 4

The Warehouse Works in Mysterious Ways

"Progress everywhere today does
seem to come so very heavily
disguised as Chaos."
-          Joyce Grenfell

As mentioned earlier, a phrase frequently used to describe operations within an Amazon FC is "organized chaos." This phraseology has even been used by Amazon itself. I can attest to the validity of this terminology since that exact feeling came to mind the minute I stepped on the warehouse floor for my day one.

The whole place was a maze of conveyor belts whizzing products around the monstrous facility at warp speed. And then there are workers everywhere zipping through the aisles pushing or pulling pallets of yellow totes and cardboard boxes. It all seemed like a blur of activity not unlike a real-life version of Pac Man.

Prior to retirement, I was in the Information Technology field for 50 or so years specializing mostly in supply chain operations from manufacturing to warehousing to distribution. I am no stranger to fulfillment centers like those in the Amazon network. As a systems analyst and software developer several decades ago, I even designed and developed inventory and warehouse management software systems for several companies. Later, when I was a high-level industry analyst for the largest IT think tank in the world, one of my specialties was evaluating the various warehouse management software systems for large corporate clients. Given this background, I am no stranger to this sector of the business world.

In the supply chain sector, a space in which Amazon is one of the largest international players, warehousing excellence can be a key differentiator often separating the winners from the losers. Many retailers, whether they be online or brick & mortar, don't actually operate their own warehouses. Some store their goods in leased warehouse space while others utilize third party logistics companies. A key to Amazon's distribution strategy is to own and operate its own warehouses, truck fleet and most of its inventory. This gives the company total control of its supply chain operations, an essential component for retailers shooting to be fast and nimble when it comes to speedy delivery and good customer service.

While owning one's warehousing space and delivery fleet is the cover charge to be a major player, excellence in fast and accurate product movement is what seals the deal. Bezos realized this from day one and invested huge quantities of time and money to get a razor-sharp competitive edge in the market.

The Need for Speed

With millions of inventory transactions occurring every day in a typical FC, Amazon realizes the need for speed. Minimizing the time it takes to receive, store, pick, pack and ship products is a key to success in the retail distribution business. Maximizing the efficiency of each of the five steps in this process is a never-ending quest in every FC.

Shaving only a second or two off the processing time of any of the five steps mentioned above funnels big bucks to the bottom line. These savings can be deployed in one of three ways: 1) reinvesting in technology and process improvements to generate more savings, 2) add to shareholder profits, or 3) reduce prices for consumers. We already know Amazon is very heavily focused on door #1. The big question is this. How much of the money flows to doors #2 and #3? The answer to that is subject to much controversy and the investigation needed to provide an answer is beyond the scope of this book.

Amazon's obsession with transaction processing speed is the primary culprit behind the company's supposed heavy-handed productivity monitoring system. While I made the point earlier in the book that workers need not worry about being fired for below average productivity, my faith in the tenacity of most American workers is restored when I see Amazonians scurrying about the warehouse to stay at the top of their game. Watching the FC "runners" moving quickly through the aisles with their pallet jacks in tow makes me think of the "running with the bulls at Pamplona," the event Hemmingway was so fond of.

Naturally, the FC runners are not really running – that would violate Amazon's strict safety policy – but they do move at quite a brisk pace. While there are the occasional slackers, it's a sight to behold during peak season.

In many traditional warehouses, storage locations for products are first determined by product type. Books go in the book section, clothing goes in the clothing section, small appliances go in their own pre-defined space, and so on. From a logical standpoint, this seems to make sense. When products arrive, workers responsible for storing products – called "stowers" in Amazon parlance – know approximately where in the warehouse each category of products should be stowed. By the same token, workers called "pickers" know approximately where to go to get items to fill customer orders.

This traditional method sounds good on the surface – "a place for everything and everything in its place." Problems begin to pop up as retail sales cycles get in the way. The space needed to store seasonal products expands and contracts on a cyclical basis. Unpredictable consumer buying patterns create haphazard space requirements as new products are continuously introduced and older products fall out of favor. Suddenly, one realizes traditional category alignment strategies result in tremendous amounts of wasted space. More storage space equates to increased "travel time" for stowing and retrieving products.

Dogfood, Diapers and D-Batteries

Like many other high-volume distributors with an incredibly diverse spectrum of products, Amazon realized that randomization of inventory locations would be needed to cut down on space requirements. At the same time, this seemingly indiscriminate storage scheme actually reduces the time needed to stow and retrieve products. Instead of the traditional "a place for everything" method mentioned above, the randomization method goes something like this, "places for anything, and everything in the most convenient place." Since the computer system keeps track of where everything is located, it can direct pickers to the best place to retrieve any given product.

Such automated placement of products randomly throughout the warehouse appears haphazard to the human eye when compared to categorized storage areas. But, the time efficiencies to be gained can be astounding. When an order picker goes to the specified location to get a case of dogfood, he or she does not have to be concerned that it may be stored right next to a large quantity of disposable diapers, flashlight batteries or whatever.

While the accuracy of computerized inventory records is of great importance to any distribution business, it is considerably more important to those using a randomized storage location strategy like Amazon's. For this reason, Amazon FCs put a great deal of emphasis on transaction accuracy. Since stowers perform the all-important first step of placing items in randomized locations, the recording of which items went into each location is an essential task in each stower's job description. While stowing productivity measured in units per hour is the most important criterion for evaluating stowers, transaction error rate comes in a close second place. FC workers must be both fast and accurate to remain in good standing.

We Don't Have No Stinking Robots

As well as reading about the supposed harsh working conditions in Amazon FCs, I also read many articles and reports exaggerating the use of automated robots to de-humanize the workforce. Some reports painted a picture of workers being forced to compete with robots as a condition of keeping their jobs. Others claimed workers were actually being supervised by robots. Nothing could be further from the truth. It's almost as if the journalists who wrote such pieces are clueless when it comes to the field of robotics.

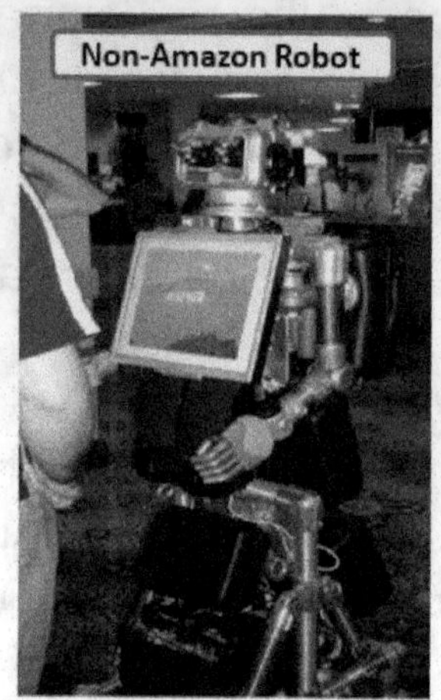

Photo Courtesy of Mike Renlund (CC BY 2.0)

Don't get me wrong. Technology gurus have made incredible breakthroughs in robotics. The human-like robots depicted in movies like *The Terminator, Transformers and Blade Runner* exist solely in the domain of the Sci-Fi thriller movies – not truly ready for prime time in the business world. Fulfillment centers consist of workers who can use their human dexterity to pick up different-sized items, examine them, stow them and pick them. Unfortunately, even the most sophisticated industrial robots still struggle with such movement. In robotics jargon, this skill is generally referred to as "grasping ability." For robots, it's not nearly as easy as it sounds.

When most people think of robotics in business, manufacturing enterprises are the first thing that comes to mind. Automated machining with things such as computer-driven cutting tools, drill presses, lathes and the like were one of the first major stages in this genre. As technology progressed, many assembly operations became automated. The automotive and high-tech electronics

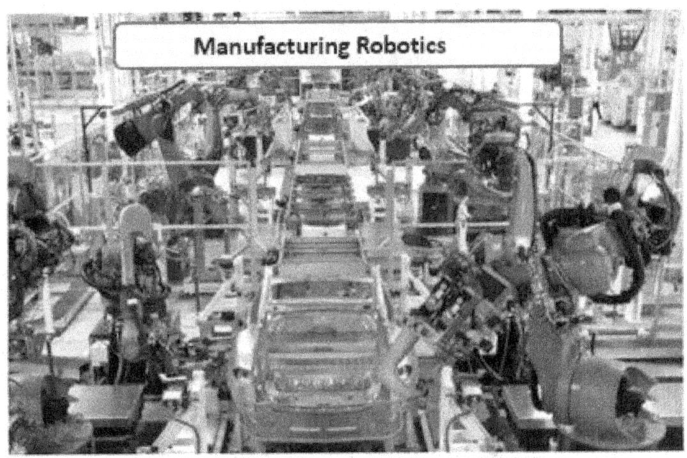

Photo Courtesy of Steve Jurvetson (CC BY 2.0)

industries were early adopters. "Lights out" operations became the mantra as designers envisioned factories run without the presence of humans.

Changing our focus from production operations to warehousing facilities, we find that manufacturers with a finite and somewhat limited number of stock-keeping units (SKUs) were the pioneers in automating warehousing operations that utilized robotics technology. The complexity and range of motion of robotics equipment used in distribution operations pale in comparison to those used in machining and assembly work.

The robotics equipment used in large warehouse operations like Amazon look nothing like those used in manufacturing. In my opinion, it's a stretch to even call them robots – because they only handle the rudimentary functions of storing and picking products in inventory. As we move into the realm of mega-warehouses where millions of items with an infinite variety of sizes and shapes need to be moved about through the warehouse, modern day robotics technology is still somewhat limited in functionality. The dexterity needed to perform the visual inspection, put-away and picking functions mentioned above is still beyond the reach (pardon the pun) of economically feasible robots. Experts agree that we are probably still a good ten years away from having robots with this functional ability.

In Amazon's heavily automated FCs, robotic equipment augments, not replaces, the work being done by humans. Used primarily in the stowing and picking functions in the warehouse, the concept is fairly simple. In traditional settings, workers push their carts around rows and aisles throughout the warehouse to do their stowing and picking to and from computer-designated shelves and bins. In Amazon FCs, the "shelves and bins" are brought to the workers' stations. In other words, so-called robots bring multi-dimensional storage bins to the workers who are assigned to individual work stations.

With the exception of very large products which are pretty much handled manually, the bulk of Amazon products are stored and moved throughout the warehouse in "pods," which are computer-controlled mobile shelving units. Each pod has two primary components: 1) a four-sided shelving unit with individual bins of different sizes, and 2) a motorized base that guides the entire unit using an intricate network of sensors in the floor of the warehouse. The shelving unit is approximately nine feet tall with each of the four sides measuring about three feet wide. Each shelving unit contains bins of differing sizes on each of its four sides. The motorized base – which essentially is the "robot" – is about three feet square and eight inches high. They look like a larger and square version of the Roomba® robot vacuum used to clean carpets in homes.

So, there you have it. Those nefarious robots taking the jobs of beleaguered Amazon warehouse workers are little more than Roombas®.

The Sequence of Events

Here's a bird's eye view of how products are processed from start to finish in fulfillment centers:

- Products arrive in large tractor-trailer and other delivery vehicles at the receiving docks.
    Most products are in large cardboard boxes that are either stacked haphazardly by themselves or in orderly fashion on pallets.

- Workers scan bar codes and sort the boxes into three receiving groups:

    1. Full pallets of identical products go to Pallet Receiving (called decanting)

    2. Products needing Amazon's manual preparation work (bagging, shrink-wrapping, etc.) go to the Prep area.
    3. All others are received individually on a Receive Line.

- Products from all three areas are removed from boxes and placed into the ubiquitous yellow totes based on size and weight parameters – maximum 25 pounds per tote.

- With input from receiving workers, the computer system keeps track of the quantities and weights of all products stored in each of the thousands of totes used to move products through downstream work stations.

- Totes are sent to the Stowing Stations to be stowed in Pods (the "robots")
  - In the newer FCs, all totes move to the stow areas on conveyer belts.
  - In older FCs, the totes and even individual cardboard cartons are moved to the stow areas on pallets by runners.

- Stowers take products from the totes and place them in storage bins in the Pods as Pods come and go to each station, automatically routed by the system.

- The automated systems use lights and sensors to record which products are stored in which Pod bin. For the semi-automated stow stations, worker input is used to record stowing transactions rather than automated sensors.

- Workers called Counters randomly tally the quantities of given products stored in each Pod bin at their Counting station as Pods are automatically routed to them.
- After customer orders are received, the system automatically routes the selected Pods to the appropriate Picking stations where pickers take the designated products from bins and place them in order picking totes.
- The order picking totes move via conveyer belt to the Pick, Pack and Ship areas adjacent to the Shipping Docks.
- If specified on the customer order, designated products are routed temporarily to a Gift Wrapping station where workers gift wrap the items.
- Shipping Pickers consolidate items by order and send them to Packing stations.
- Individual products or multiple products for a single order are packed for shipping.
  - Depending on size, weight and shape, certain products can be packed by automated packing machines while others are packed manually by workers.
- Products packaged in Amazon boxes are loaded into trucks at the shipping docks.

The last step in the process is of course the whisking away of products in Amazon delivery trucks and third-party delivery service vehicles.

Taking It to the Streets – FBA Style

Never let a good idea go to waste. That has been one of my mantras over the years as an entrepreneur. In fact, I've taken the concept to an even higher level in my belief and practice that good ideas should be expanded, exploited and implemented with great passion. A few of my personal brainstorms fizzled due to inadequate follow-through or lack of adequate funding, but several of those I took to fruition made me lots of money. Amazon capitalized on this concept to double the size of its business, making my personal efforts seem like child's play.

In following Amazon's expansion in warehousing and distribution over the years, I see two pivotal strategic ideas that fueled the company's phenomenal growth to become the world's largest retailer. The first is well known to almost everyone and that was Bezos' strategy from the beginning to expand well beyond the brilliant concept of an online bookstore. He did this by building an incredibly sturdy business foundation and then leveraging the hell out of it. That one is already in the business history books.

The second strategic idea that had as much impact but may not have been in mind at the company's launch happened around 2001. This was seven years after the inception of Amazon. Rather than only selling its own inventory, I imagine the thought in Bezos head went something like this. "Since we're building the 900-pound gorilla in the retail sales and distribution arena, why not offer those services to other manufacturers and distributors and charge them handsome fees for doing so. Now that eBay has proven the business model, we can do the same thing only bigger, better and faster."

Voila! Fulfillment by Amazon (FBA) was born. The service provides storage, packaging, and shipping assistance to sellers. Those three necessary functions can be time-consuming and expensive distractions for businesses and entrepreneurs, especially those just getting started. Amazon's expertise gives the company the economies of scale that leave others in the dust economically. Add to the pure financial numbers Amazon's ultra-speedy delivery services and you might say it's a match made in heaven. Faster than Domino's® Pizza? Hardly – but perhaps the fastest non-pizza delivery service available.

The FBA program allows sellers to ship their merchandise to an Amazon fulfillment center, where items are stored in warehouses until they are sold. Amazon enforces specific requirements for certain products such as leak-proof sealing, poly bagging and bubble wrapping. Sellers can choose to have Amazon do this preparation for a per-item fee and that prep work is performed in the FC as part of the receiving process. When an order is placed, Amazon employees physically pick, package, and ship the goods, after which the seller is billed.

Having the Amazon name associated with their products give sellers a marketing edge over their competitors. It establishes a high level of trust with consumers who expect good customer service and rapid, dependable delivery. Because Amazon has its own delivery fleet and a solid relationship with many shipping companies, sellers using FBA may even save money on delivery costs. From a marketing standpoint, sellers can offer free shipping over a certain dollar amount since products sold through FBA are eligible for Amazon Prime free shipping.

Sellers can offer their products through Amazon's online marketplace or on their own website with the FBA logo. In either case, Amazon does the "heavy lifting" of fulfillment. Fees charged for the FBA service can be costly, however, with Amazon taking typically 15%-18% in fees on each sale. Good for Amazon but maybe not so good for sellers. Storage fees can accumulate quickly for slow-moving or oversized products. Sellers are also charged removal fees for defective, damaged, and unsellable products.

Part of Amazon's "organized chaos" scenario allows products to be commingled regardless of who owns each specific item in the shared warehouse space. Even though the exact same product may be mixed together with others regardless of ownership, Amazon's sophisticated computer system knows the difference and handles the financial transactions accordingly.

One often unanticipated downside for sellers comes from Amazon's very generous, no-questions-asked return policy. This guarantees buyers free return privileges if not satisfied. Once customers catch on to how easy it is to return products bought from Amazon, the number of returned products naturally goes up. I can attest to this

> **It's no wonder that Fulfillment By Amazon sales make up over half of total company retail sales**

from personal experience as an Amazon customer. If I'm uncertain about the size of an article of clothing I'm buying for instance, I might order it in two sizes. When they arrive, I keep the one that fits best and return the other for free with a full refund. UPS will even pick up the returned item as part of the service.

One great thing about the FBA program is its one-size-fits-all deployment. Whether you're a multi-million dollar manufacturer or a mom-and-pop sole proprietor business, you can make FBA work for you. This is not Amazon marketing hype, it's my expert opinion as a successful marketer. I not only sell my books on the Amazon marketplace, but I self-published all my books using Amazon's publishing subsidiary, Kindle Publishing. It's no wonder that FBA sales make up over half of total company retail sales.

The Cardboard Jungle

It did not take me long after I started work to realize one staggering reality. Amazon FCs handle more cardboard than almost any other business on earth. While I used my well-honed research skills in an attempt to snare some actual numbers on cardboard use, I found it impossible to come up with a valid number for Amazon.

There are two huge components to the cardboard box game plan – incoming and outgoing. Working in the Receiving department, I saw personally the humongous volume of incoming cardboard boxes from all the vendors shipping products to Amazon for sale. While I did not work on the shipping side of the business, I couldn't help but notice the hundreds of pallets of shipping boxes being queued up for packing of outgoing orders.

According to an article I read on mrboxonline.com, I learned Amazon ships over 600 million packages each year. That's a hell of a lot of cardboard, and that's only on the outgoing side.

Having worked for one of the world's largest forest products companies many moons ago, my educated guess is that Amazon probably sells its used incoming cardboard box carcasses to paper mills to be used in pulp production.

One essential machine center in all FCs is the cardboard compactor that crushes and compacts used cardboard into bales to be recycled. If you question my word "essential," picture this. The compactor appears to be a maintenance-sensitive piece of equipment that needs constant care and attention. Every time the compactor jams, the empty cardboard box conveyer belt comes to a halt. While a team of mechanics and engineers scramble to get it operating again, workers at the many receiving and prep stations are quickly overrun by the heavy volume of cardboard boxes.

It does not take much time for receiving stations to start drowning in a sea of cardboard. Enter the runners who pull recycling pallets to each of the receiving stations. On each pallet is a huge blue cardboard bin measuring about five feet square and six feet high. The incoming shipping boxes tend to be on the large size, so these bins fill up quickly and the team of runners stays busy hauling bins to and from the stations.

The recycling pallets are taken to special elevators that take the castaway cardboard up several floors to the compacting area. As you can surmise, when the compactor machinery is shut down for a lengthy period, the upper floor itself becomes inundated with more cardboard then can be handled. And, you guessed it, the elevator must cease operation until the compactor is brought back online.

I vividly recall one ill-fated week in which the cardboard compactor was down for four straight days. The entire Receiving area became a cardboard jungle. Recycling bins were tucked away in every nook and cranny available after they consumed enormous chunks of floor space. Aisles were crammed full of the big blue bins. Productivity slowed to a near crawl as people spent excessive amounts of time looking for unused storage space. From a management perspective, it was a nightmare. I can still remember the clapping and cheering when the cardboard conveyer belt fired back into operation.

From Cardboard Boxes to Computer Bugs

Less visible than the cardboard compactor meltdown, the intermittent computer glitches caused their own nightmares, Well, perhaps nightmare is an overstatement. They were more like bad dreams that interrupt a good night's sleep. The nefarious nature of computer bugs is that they are often inconsistent and therefore hard to detect and even harder to fix. Then of course there's the electronic finger-pointing. It's a hardware problem... no, it's a software malfunction. It's often hard to tell which.

From my many years in the IT field, I'm certainly no stranger to computer glitches. Some are caused by faulty data input that was undetected by failsafe protections such as data integrity filters. Then of course there are the occasional hardware failures that are especially hard to pin down if they are intermittent. Software bugs are usually the most frustrating since re-creating an error incident caused by a given set of seemingly mysterious circumstances can be an exercise in futility.

As a software developer many years ago, I became pretty adept at spotting, investigating and fixing bugs in software. Back in the day, I developed a reputation of being somewhat of a Sherlock Holmes of software malfunction investigations. I recall some nights running test after test until sunrise before I finally tracked down the unique series of events that caused a bug to surface. The only reason for me pointing that out is to highlight the fact that I have a trained eye when it comes to spotting software bugs. The more sophisticated the software, the more likely that bugs exist…and the harder they will be to detect.

So, what does all this have to do with my Amazon FC experience? Thanks. I'm glad you brought that up.

 I've already touched on the fact that the software used to control and monitor operations within an FC is highly complex. The hardware and software used to track productivity statistics and highlight operator errors is especially concerning in the stowing operation. This is due primarily to the complexities inherent with computerized sensors and multicolored lighting indicators.

Putting on my computer software developer hat, my professional opinion is that the software in use in Amazon FCs is lightly infected with undetected bugs. Is this situation highly problematic? My realistic answer is a definite no. Having said that it can be annoying and can lead to disagreement between front-line workers and managers.

While I never got into any serious confrontations with FC managers, I was admonished a few times in situations where they smugly pointed out errors I supposedly made. In their infinite wisdom, they blindly adhere to the assumption that the system is infallible and the worker is dreadfully error prone. No logical argument will ever change their mind on this.

Real People Make a Difference

In my research activities, I read many accounts of employee dissatisfaction with working conditions at various FCs around the country. When I read about guys whining because it is physically devastating to work at Amazon, I think about all the petite women who work tirelessly at the PDX9 FC with few complaints. One woman in particular stands out as an example. While I worked on the receiving dock, I had the pleasure of working side by side with a lady I'll call Ms. Flowers. I don't want to use her real name as this story might come back to haunt her.

While Ms. Flowers is in her mid-40s and weighs in at about 100 pounds like the petite females I mentioned earlier, she is as tough as nails when it comes to her job. She has arthritis in her hands and joints but you'd never know it when you watch her work. Flowers once had me work with her on an assignment to muscle 1,800-pound pallets around the warehouse for re-positioning. I fancy myself as being pretty strong, but it was all I could do to keep up with her pace. Pardon the Humphry Bogart language but she is one tough broad

I heard lots of guys complaining about having to lift 40-50 pound boxes of product even though that's what they agreed to when they applied for the job. Amazon puts that job requirement right up front when they advertise job openings. Ms. Flowers, on the other hand, stacked heavy boxes for hours on end as she handled pallet loads of incoming products on the receiving dock.

Then I also think of Mohammed, a wiry kid from Malaysia who was partially crippled by polio in his youth and still walks with a prominent limp. I've never seen a frown on Mohammed's face. Rather than sit around and complain about the physical limitations life has handed him, he does his best to keep up with his physically fit co-workers.

Chapter 5

The Job of the Associate

"In the middle of difficulty lies
opportunity"
- Albert Einstein

In the previous chapter, I explained my view of how a typical Amazon fulfillment center (FC) works. Here, I'll drop down to a more granular level and get into the various jobs Amazon warehouse workers – excuse me, "associates" – perform their day-to-day activities. Keep in mind that since I only actually worked in the front-end receiving departments at PDX9, I am not fully versed at jobs in other areas. For this information, I had to piece together what I had heard in conversations with workers from other areas of the building.

Also keep in mind as you're reading my story about working in an Amazon FC the fact that my wants and desires were different than others who work there. Being fairly well off financially, I was certainly not doing it for the money. But you already knew that simply from the title of the book. Most of my co-workers were there because they needed a job to put food on the table and a roof over their heads. I tried to keep that different perspective squarely in mind as I compiled these pages.

Keeping that caveat in mind, information I'm sharing here about specific jobs within the FC may be second hand, which means accuracy may not be 100%. Also be aware that PDX9 where I worked may operate differently than other FCs around the country, much less, around the globe. This is not due to a lack of standardization but to the fact that the various FC facilities are growing and changing constantly. This causes them to be in different stages of maturity when it comes to technology and processes. Thirdly, you should understand that my goal as stated in the title of this book colors my outlook about working conditions. That being the case, many of my comments will be made in the context of how much and what kind of physical exercise is typically involved in each job description. If you're reading this book to help you make a decision on whether or not to pursue employment at an FC facility, I hope this will aid in your decision making.

In the course of my research leading up to my applying for work at Amazon, I read lots of bogus tales of deplorable working conditions and poverty-level employment. I found much of what I read to be gross exaggeration interspersed with vicious lies. While my starting wage was the company standard of $15 per hour, I was pleased to see that by the end of my first year, my pay had risen to almost $17 per hour plus a few bonuses. If you plug that into your calculator, you'll see that comes to a little over $35,000 per year – and that's before the overtime money paid during peak season in the fourth quarter. Anything over 40 hours per week pays $25.50 per hour or $255 per day. By my calculation, if one works an average of a little more than 1

½ overtime days a month, total annual income exceeds $40 grand. With all that, I never asked for a raise. I found pay increases to be virtually automatic regardless of effort expended or quotas met. So, that pretty much blows the top off the lie that Amazon pays slave wages which are below the poverty line. Shame on you journalists.

One important thing I must point out at this juncture is that newly hired employees almost never have the luxury of choosing which specific jobs they will be handed after they are hired. That is based on the particular FC's needs at the time of hire. In general, most applicants are looking only at the job title "warehouse associate."

Here's a tip for all of you potential job seekers who are reading this. Regardless of the specific job you get assigned to on day one, try to do the best job you can with the tasks you are handed. Being in the good graces of your first boss and other nearby supervisors will increase your chances of being reassigned to jobs more to your liking. Once you start working, be observant of activities that are going on around you, specifically in nearby departments.

Strike up conversations with co-workers, especially in the breakrooms and ask lots of questions about the different kinds of jobs others are doing. This will help you target the jobs most appealing to your skills and goals. Don't be afraid to discuss your job description preferences with your boss and associated supervisors. Typically, they won't take your comments in a negative light. One general theme within the FC workplace is that cross-training for other jobs within the FC is welcomed because it increases the flexibility of the overall workforce. Personally, I always gladly accepted opportunities to try new job duties even if I was not too wild about the tasks involved.

The extra effort I put forth and the flexibility I demonstrate is greatly appreciated by the management team in my current area and they recognize me for it regularly. Of course, I had worked in a different area for a few months prior to that and the approach there was not as worker-friendly. Managers and supervisors in that area gave all their attention to the productivity statistics and no other factors seemed to matter to them. It was therefore, a more hostile environment but still not as bad as the accounts I had read in the media.

At the risk of putting some of you to sleep with talk of statistics, there is one statistical term I must share with you because it comes up a lot in conversation with FC workers, especially in a few specific jobs. The term "takt time" comes from the German word for cycle time and refers to the amount of time it takes to process a unit of goods through a work step. This definition will become much clearer in the contexts used below.

A word of caution for anyone taking a job in an Amazon warehouse who needs personal recognition: you probably won't get it here. I do want to stress the word "probably" because I saw several exceptions to the rule, especially in the Receiving area. In my view, most of the managers and supervisors are so busy managing the inherent chaos and striving to meet their quotas, they simply don't have time to give pep talks or dispense kudos. Welcome to the proletariat world. If you need heartfelt encouragement, you'd better get it at home before you come to work. That sounds harsh, but you'll most likely not get any "touchy feely" reassurance in manual labor environments such as Amazon FCs.

Big Brother Is Always Watching

Sorry if I burst your bubble with my last dose of reality and it won't get any better in this paragraph. One thing to be aware of when working in an Amazon warehouse is that there are cameras everywhere. This is not some sinister plot on the part of the company but mostly a precautionary measure. Surveillance cameras are so inexpensive these days that most large companies use them extensively, but spying on employees is not a primary objective.

Industrial accidents are not uncommon in manual labor workplaces, especially those heavily automated. When it comes to investigating causes of accidents in the workplace, video camera footage can prove invaluable.

Beyond that, video taping of workers performing their jobs can be quite a boon to management when it comes to determining needs for training and re-training. Personally, I have no objection to any employer taping my on-the-job activities. I do not see it as an invasion of my privacy. After all, the company is paying me to do a job and that pretty much gives them the right to make sure I'm doing it correctly.

I did have one particular incident happen that I feel I should share with you. One day, I was simply going about my duties as a stower when suddenly a message popped up on my workstation screen. Basically, it said, "Keep in mind that when something falls out of a bin and onto the floor, you're responsible." Since a product had just fallen to the floor from one of the bins on a pod I was working, it certainly got my attention. "Son-of-a bitch," I thought as I looked around. "How did they jump on that so fast?" I had to chuckle as I realized they were watching on camera. Oh well, no harm, no foul I realized. The item was not broken and I was not reprimanded. I had to smile as I pictured my supervisor laughing when he saw my reaction to the message he sent.

There was another incident that happened on a different day, also in the stow area. Again, I was going about my duties and fighting off the boredom of the job. I became rather annoyed by the folks in the station next to mine. Do note that "folks" is plural. I point this out since there is only one worker per station mostly all day long.

What was going on next door to me was a stark exception to that rule. Three co-workers, two girls and one guy, would gather intermittently throughout the shift for some intense gossip and idle chatter. It went on for hours. The constant yapping and laughing was getting on my nerves. Why were they allowed to get away with this? Why was no one watching on camera? Why were there no managers or safety people walking past our stations? I wrote it off to being a slow Sunday afternoon and tried to put the distraction out of my mind.

Job-by-job Breakdown

I'll list these jobs in a somewhat random sequence covering the ones I'm familiar with from personal experience first and then moving on to the others. Almost all jobs require workers to be on their feet for almost all of the ten or eleven hour shift. By order of importance, the three biggest jobs are stow, pick and pack. The majority of new hires end up in one of those three jobs, with stow being at the top of the heap.

Stower – workers who stow products in pods

At PDX9, the stow area spanned vertically through four floors and is by far the largest area within the FC. Since it is typically the area to which most new hires are assigned, it serves as sort of a boot camp for the majority of FC associates. Almost all of the negative stories I researched in the media centered around complaints made by stowers. Stowing is one of the most stringently measured processes in every FC. In the stow area, the expected takt time is 12 seconds. In other words, a stower is expected to pick up a product, pass it by the scanner and place it in a properly sized bin in a pod every 12 seconds. That equates to ten products every two minutes.

Expected takt time measurements are of course the averages achieved over periods of time such as "units per hour." It may take a stower less than 5 seconds on average per unit to stow a case of small aspirin bottles. But what about 16-pound cases of dog food? Bulky items naturally take longer to stow mostly because fitting them into a bin is more difficult than fitting in a bottle of aspirin. I realize this seems like a miner point to most of you readers, but it can easily become a heated argument between workers and managers in the FC. To realize the full impact of this seemingly minor point, you must realize that supervisors and managers are held to similar expectations when higher level managers are measuring them based on average takt time for their crews and departments.

Computer controlled colored lights are used to illuminate "off limit" bins once the stower passes an item over a scanner. After determining which item is about to be stowed based on the item number just scanned, the system knows which bins in the pod are unacceptable for stowing the given product. It may be that the item is similar to one or more already stowed in the bin. For instance, large size red T-shirts should not be in a bin already containing size medium red T-shirts. We'll see later that this will make the picker's job tougher.

One thing to remember when talking about metrics such as takt time is that the "average" times include ancillary tasks. Such steps involve visually eyeballing each arriving pod looking for open bin space large enough to stow the products at hand, manipulating hard to manage packaging to make barcodes readable and discarding empty cardboard boxes as they are emptied. And don't forget that since the pods are nine feet tall, it can mean moving up and down a ladder to reach the higher bins. All in all, it can be a taxing exercise to keep up with takt time expectations.

Personally, I did not find the stowing job, which I did for over two months straight, to be overly taxing from a physical standpoint. I did find it incredibly boring, however, and often could hardly wait until my shift was over.

From a physical exercise standpoint, the stow job is moderate for both aerobic exercise and muscle building.

Water Spider – workers who keep stowers supplied with items to stow

Borrowed from the manufacturing sector, this odd-sounding term refers to a person tasked with keeping workstations fully stocked with materials, thus controlling the continuous flow of productivity. This is fast and furious work that is perhaps the most physically demanding job in the FC. Water spiders scurry around pulling pallets of totes and boxes from elevator bays to the workstations. They must lift the totes and boxes from the pallets and place them on roller belts that feed each stower's work table (called a sled).

Since some products are sold as individual items and others are sold by the box, it is the water spider who must decide whether or not to open boxes of products as they load them onto the sleds. They must scan the box labels to make that decision. Wrong decisions can cause serious errors that affect productivity and customer service.

Water spider productivity is not measured on positive metrics like takt time. They are judged based on the avoidance of negatives:

- Number of "Low on Work" or "Out of Work" incidents at stow stations
- Number of box opening errors – individual vs. carton stowing

From a physical exercise standpoint, the water spider job gives workers a high level of both aerobic exercise and muscle building.

Receiver – Logs incoming products into the system

Workers in the Receiving department process incoming products in two ways – individual receiving or pallet load receiving (called decanting). For individual receiving, products arrive at receiver stations via conveyer belt. As the name implies, products acceptable for pallet load receiving arrive…you guessed it, in full pallets. For pallet load receiving, pallets must contain products that are all identical. On the individual receiving line on the other hand, boxes may arrive that may contain a mix of different products.

The photo shows me receiving several cartons of dumbbells. I grab any opportunity I can for a little extra weight training.

As products are logged into the computer system as being received and ready for sale, workers remove them from boxes and load them into totes based on size and weight. Totes cannot contain more than 25 pounds of products and the height of product(s) cannot come any closer than one inch from the top of the tote. This allows totes to be stacked in a nested fashion.

From a physical exercise standpoint, muscle exertion depends on the size and weight of the individual products. Bars of soap naturally do not require receivers to work up a sweat, but 12-pound jugs of laundry detergent are a different story. I once received a 5,000 pound pallet of barbell weights. I definitely needed a break when I finished that task, which required over an hour.

Problem Solver – Brains over Brawn

Problem solver workers can be found across several departments throughout the FC with most of the problems needing solutions occurring in the Receiving and Stowing areas. These folks each have a cart on which sits their laptop computer, a label printer and a small assortment of supplies. The online computer is used to research conditions that appear to be in error like missing or invalid bar codes, improper packaging that leads to counting errors (like individual vs. bulk), items that need prep before being officially received as ready to stow, products not properly labeled and things of that nature.

From a physical exercise standpoint, problem solver jobs almost never involve physical exertion, but they are not for couch potatoes either. Like most other FC associates, they are on their feet all day long.

Down-stacker – Wheaties for breakfast may be required

At the end of conveyer belts coming from the Receive Line, you'll find lots of heavy lifting going on that looks and feels like a good hard workout at the gym…and it is just as taxing. As full totes weighing up to 30 pounds each come rocketing down the line, the mighty down-stackers keep busy lifting them off the line and stacking them onto pallets. Totes are stacked five high on the pallets which hold 30 totes each.

From a physical exercise standpoint, down-stackers do heavy lifting for hours on end. Thirty pounds may not sound like a lot of weight, but when you're stacking them on the top layer of a 5-layer-high pallet, it can wear you out fast. The meeker associates avoid the down-stacking area for fear they will be pressed into service. I have a special tank top emblazoned with the phrase "I Lift Heavy Shit" that I enjoy wearing on my down-stacking shifts.

Runner – Actually, fast walker

A well-established staple of the FC is the runner. They're everywhere, especially during peak times. They may be pushing pallets of product or giant receptacles of empty cardboard boxes seemingly at warp speed from point A to point B in the warehouse. Or they may be Tote Runners pushing large platform carts holding over a hundred empty totes to be dropped off at picking or receiving stations. These carts are called Tanks because of their ominous girth and you do not want to get in their way.
From a physical exercise standpoint, runners get a ton of aerobic exercise. Depending on workload, runners who multi-task with down-stacking chores also get plenty of heavy lifting added to their regimen.

Counter – Confirms and/or corrects bin inventory quantities

Quite possibly the most mind-numbing and isolated job in the FC, the counter works in solitude counting the quantities of the various items stowed in the pod bins. These pods are automatically routed to the counting stations. The spectrum of different product sizes is enormous ranging from 25-pound boat anchors to tiny pieces of jewelry weighing in at less than an ounce. Needless to say, patience and laser-like attention to detail are essential skills here. Since the system tracks what supposedly went into each bin along with time and worker ID stamps, stowing errors can be tracked back to individual workers…at least that's the logical assumption. Since I was never accused of errors involving quantity counts, I'm not sure that assumption is valid. I was accused, however, of a few stowing transgressions that involved "overstuffed bins."

Bin overstuffing occurs when stowers become too aggressive in cramming as many units into a bin as possible. This is an example of situations where undue attention given to metrics such as takt times can be a little counterproductive. Feeling the pressure to achieve low takt times, I packed some bins really tight. While bins typically looked OK as the pods left my station, the constant jarring of pods as they are propelled to and fro through the warehouse can shake some products loose. This may cause them to hang outside the confines of the bin. Oops! As I was being warned of my overstuffing sins, I was shown incriminating photos of said bins with the date, time and my employee number stamped on them. My assumption is that these photos are taken at counter stations. "Mea Culpa, I promise never to overstuff again. But remember, this will negatively affect my takt times."

From a physical exercise standpoint, counters burn close to zero calories and get no physical exercise except for finger movement as they count sequentially through hundreds of greeting cards occasionally. That was a joke, BTW.

Auditors – FC "policemen" who enforce the rules and issue tickets to violators

While auditors don't arrive with red lights flashing, they do arrive with laptops open. Laptop screens have proof of a rule violation such as receiving a quantity of a given item that exceeded the number of items ordered. Bam! Violators are usually "written up" for their transgressions and get the corresponding black mark on their record. These black marks can mean employee requests for things such as job or shift transfers may be rejected or they can even lead to termination.

From a physical exercise standpoint, auditors burn close to zero calories and get no physical exercise other than occasionally jumping to conclusions.

Picker – takes from pods, puts in large totes, sends to Outbound

Order Pickers perform the mirror function of stowers but their workstations look essentially the same. Rather than traversing warehouse aisles looking for the designated items to grab and place in their "shopping carts" like traditional pickers, Amazon order pickers remain at fixed workstations. Computer controlled pods are routed electronically to the picking stations where light beams point to the bins in which the ordered products are stored. From several products available in the illuminated bin, the picker selects the proper item(s) and passes them by the scanner. Remember than due to randomized storage, dogfood and D-batteries may be in the same bin. The scanner beeps a warning if the selected item is incorrect.

The picker places the item(s) in the tote designated by the system. To minimize overall average picking time, items from multiple orders may end up in a particular tote. That will be addressed later. When directed by the system, the picker will push specific totes on the outbound conveyer belt which routes them to the outbound side of the FC.

From a physical exercise standpoint, the picker job is very similar to the stower job. It is moderate for both aerobic exercise and muscle building.

Trailer unloader – Moves products from trucks to receiving dock

There are basically two methods used for unloading trailers – by forklift or manually. Forklift unloading can only be done if products are neatly stacked on pallets and these pallets are most often taken to the pallet receiving area, referred to as the decanting line. When unloading non-palletized goods, workers must scan the various labels on each box of goods to determine the next step. FBA products requiring preparation by Amazon workers are routed to the prep area while others are staged for single case receiving. There is a third routing possibility. Cases that cannot be clearly identified are given to problem solvers for disposition.

From a physical exercise standpoint, the manual unloader job is one of the most taxing due to heavy lifting. It can be back-breaking work but definitely not aerobic exercise. Unloaders using forklifts need more skill but less muscle power.

Order Inductors – located on the outbound side of the FC, inductors process large totes arriving on conveyer belts from order picking.

After each incoming tote and its contents are scanned, individual products are moved to small totes that are sent down the line toward the packing section. These small totes may contain a single item or several identical items for a given order.

From a physical exercise standpoint, inductors get a moderate amount of physical lifting exercise but no aerobic exercise worth mentioning.

Re-bin Operators – from small totes to cubby hole bins

As the small totes arrive at the re-bin station, items are scanned and workers are directed to a computer assign order bin where each individual item is to be placed. Light sensors indicate when all items for the order are in the order bin. The re-bin operator then pushes the order bin through to the other side of the wall signaling the order is complete and ready to ship.

From a physical exercise standpoint, re-bin operators get a medium dose of aerobic exercise, perhaps even a heavy dose during peak times. Physical lifting exercise is typically moderate.

**Packers – Not to be mistaken for football players
from Green Bay, they pack boxes**

On the packing side of the outbound wall, packers put items in boxes with the proper amount of packing material. Packers do not have to determine proper box sizes because the computer does that for them. Full boxes go to the Slam machine, where a shipping label is "slammed" on the box and the box is sealed automatically.

From a physical exercise standpoint, Amazon packers get light doses of both aerobic and lifting exercise.

**Truck loader – Load boxes of product into trailers
and other delivery vehicles**

Here's where the rubber is about to meet the road. Computers, sensors and conveyor belts route boxes by zip code to the appropriate doors on the shipping dock where loaders put them in the proper vehicles for final delivery.

From a physical exercise standpoint, this is one of the most demanding jobs in the FC for both aerobic and lifting exercise. Things really get frantic during peak times as workers must continually play the FC game of "beat the clock." The clock for each order starts when the computer receives the order. From that point, FC workers have 48 hours to pick, induct, re-bin, pack, slam, sort and ship each order.

Safety Specialists – Similar to auditors, the safety "police persons" watch for safety violations

Often wearing green vests, the roaming (or sometimes standing) safety specialists move through the facility reminding workers of safety precautions, such as where they cannot sit during breaks. The 2020 pandemic probably caused a doubling or tripling of safety workers tasked with ensuring proper mask wearing, social distancing and similar precautions.

From a physical exercise standpoint, roaming safety workers get plenty of walking exercise, while those on stationary assignments get little or none.

Working Hours

If you're looking for a 4-day work week, an Amazon FC is one place you'll find that. It's nice having 3-day weekends, but there's a hitch. Those three days may be in the middle of the week, and ten-hour days can be a little grueling, especially if you're in one of the more physically demanding jobs outlined above. Plus, keep in mind that during peak times like from Thanksgiving through Christmas, eleven-hour workdays are pretty much mandatory. Having said that, I was surprised to find out how easy Amazon makes it to "get around" those supposedly mandatory overtime hours. Within stated guidelines, the options associates have for adjusting their own work hours can be quite nice at times.

As to which of the seven days of a work week each individual associate must work, there are three basic patterns: 1) Sunday through Wednesday, 2) Thursday through Sunday, and 3) Monday, Tuesday, Thursday and Friday. Those of course are for full time workers. Part time work can be either fixed schedule or flex time, the latter of which can be quite flexible as the name implies. Fixed schedule part timers are generally scheduled for 20 hours per week. Flex time workers can go online and see which days and time periods - , mornings, afternoons or night shifts – are available each week. Once a worker signs up for a shift, it is considered mandatory for them.

All other work hour options are designated by 3-letter acronyms:

VAC – Vacation Time
Full-time associates earn about 1 ½ hours of vacation time per week starting out. That comes to 40 hours per year in year one. In year two, it goes up to 80 hours and increments from there. Vacation time can be accrued up to a maximum of 160 hours. VAC can only be used with 24-hour advance notice and cannot be used during peak season.

PTO – Personal Time Off
Each full-time associate earns PTO hours each week based on the number of hours worked that week. However, the maximum number of PTO hours that can be earned is capped at 48 hours per year. New employees are given 10 hours of PTO on day one. PTO can be used anytime without giving prior notice, even during the peak season.

UPT – Unpaid Time
A novel feature of Amazon's compensation program is the UPT allocation. When employees are out of or don't want to use VAC or PTO, they can utilize UPT with the

understanding that it's unpaid time off. New hires get 10 hours of UPT to be used at their discretion. After that, each employee receives 20 hours of UPT each calendar quarter. A maximum of 80 hours of UPT can be accrued with unused hours rolled over to the next year. UPT can be used anytime and no approval is necessary. If a worker leaves before the end of shift and no PTO is used, UPT will be taken from his or her allocation automatically. The only downside is that when a person's UPT hits zero, that person is typically terminated immediately.

MET – Mandatory Extra Time (Overtime)
Used primarily during peak season, MET can be mandated by management. MET can be designated in hours or days. A regular 10-hour shift can be extended by one or two hours. When workload is exceptionally heavy, management can mandate an extra full shift to be added to the work week. Employees are notified in advance by text and/or email of upcoming MET requirements. At each employee's discretion, PTO or UPT can be used to offset the additional MET if he or she has such available.

VET – Voluntary Extra Time
During times of heavy workload, managers can offer VET opportunities to employees who want to earn some extra cash. The opportunities can be found on the Amazon employee portal. These extra shifts or half-shifts are strictly voluntary, but once an employee signs up to take a VET opportunity, that shift becomes mandatory.

VTO – Voluntary Time Off
On days when the workload is lighter than anticipated, VTO can be offered on a first come, first served basis. Upcoming VTO opportunities can be found on the Amazon

employee portal or can be offered to employees verbally during regular shifts. While VTO is unpaid time off, the hours are not deducted for accrued UPT allocations.

As one can see from the assortment of working days and hours options, Amazon warehouse workers most likely have more flexibility than most other similar jobs in other companies. Amazon makes it easy for workers to move to other positions or departments simply by entering requests on the employee Internet portal. So, why all the bitching by disgruntled employees and journalists?

Personally, I feel that the flexibility offered in FC jobs coupled with the above average wages paid make Amazon warehouses pretty good places to work. Note, I did not say great, but good overall. I talked to many co-workers who were happy to be employed there. That's a far cry from all the doom and gloom pitched by some disenchanted ex-employees and the media.

Internal Job Hopping

Still not enough flexibility for you? Another nice feature of working for Amazon is the scope of its internal job transfer offering. The revolving door caused by high employee turnover coupled with the explosive growth rate of the company offers yet another flexibility pathway. Internally, Amazon has a somewhat robust job transfer system. Don't like the job you have? Request a different one. Don't like the shift or hours you work? Request a different work pattern.

The internal job transfer mechanism is housed on the Internet-based employee portal. Employees can go to the portal and browse available jobs, shifts and working hour patterns available at their own location or any other Amazon location. When one finds an opportunity they like, he or she simply requests the transfer online. Open requests are reviewed continuously and job transfers are granted at least once a month. Transferees are retrained for their new job so no experience is required. All that's necessary is that the employee has a clean record, which means no current infractions.

Chapter 6

Benefits Beyond Better Health

"People work for money, but they
go the extra mile for recognition,
praise and rewards."
-    Dale Carnegie

The value of employee benefits is an often-overlooked part of a worker's true compensation. I like to refer to them as soft wages since they provide a financial cushion on which many workers rely but seldom give their employers credit for providing. Healthcare benefits is an area that has been bandied about for the past several years and people get very emotional when arguing about whether it's a human right or a privilege to be earned. I'll step out on a limb here and state openly I'm on the earned privilege side of the issue. Is free healthcare mentioned in the Bill of Rights? No. Or even the Constitution? Nope. If healthcare is a right, who thought up the idea of imposing a deductible? And why would there be a need for one?

I am steadfastly against government provided healthcare after seeing the negative economic effects this concept has had on the economies of other countries. Our Canadian neighbors to the great white north can attest to that…eh? Everything the government touches turns into a very expensive political mess. Common logic has proven the Social Security system is little more than a Ponzi scheme. Agencies such as the Veterans Affairs and DMV have become bureaucratic labyrinths. If you want something to be priced at twice as much as it's worth, make it part of the government. Why then would we trust the government to be in charge of our healthcare?

But, I digress – sorry for getting off topic. Just wanted you to know where my mindset rests on one particular aspect of employee benefits.

I want to get into the subject of employee benefits provided to Amazon warehouse workers. In my travels, I've experienced healthcare benefits provided by a wide array of organizations so this isn't my first rodeo. While I've certainly seen other employee benefits packages much more attractive than those provided at Amazon FCs, I've also seen many that don't come close to measuring up to what Amazon provides.

You'll see from the following dissertation, that I have more positive feelings about Amazon FC benefits than negative ones. Like other opinions I state in this book, I want to stress these are my opinions and in no way meant to be neither an advertisement *for*, nor an indictment *of* Amazon. I'm certainly neutral on the healthcare benefits issue since the combination of government provided Medicare coverage (which by itself is very weak) and private coverage in the form of Medicare Advantage (which is quite strong) surpasses what Amazon offers. But that observation applies only to retirees like me.

Overall, Amazon provides a wide range of benefits to regular, full-time U.S. employees, eligible family members, domestic partners and their children. I'll try to stay out of the weeds, so here's the *Reader's Digest* version.

Healthcare

Medical, prescription drug, dental and vision coverage are available. Costs and deductibles are what I'd call average when compared to what other organizations provide. One nice aspect of Amazon's plans is that they kick in on day one with no waiting period to begin coverage.

Employees can choose from several plans, including multiple network providers and a health savings account option with employee and employer contributions. Associates can also enroll in dental and vision plans as well as government approved flexible spending accounts.

Company Paid Insurance

Amazon pays for basic Life and Accidental Death & Dismemberment Insurance with the option to enroll in additional coverage for the employee and dependents. There is also company-paid Short-Term and Long-Term Disability insurance.

401(k) Deferred Income Savings Plan

Amazon's 401(k) plan allows employees to defer income tax free for long-term savings and does match employee contributions up to 4%. The plan offers a variety of investment options to help you reach your financial goals.

Maternity, Parental and Adoption Leave

Amazon offers a range of fully paid maternity and parental Leave options for parents prior to, and following, the birth or adoption of a child. The company includes a "leave share" option and a flexible return-to-work program known as "Ramp Back." Parental options require at least one year of continuous service by the date of a child's birth or adoption placement.

The company offers up to 20 weeks of leave to birth mothers and six weeks for parents who adopt. The leave share program allows employees to give six weeks of paid parental leave to a spouse or partner who isn't eligible for parental leave from their employer. The Ramp Back program offers birth parents eight consecutive weeks of flexibility and partial work hours as they readjust to work schedules.

Employee Assistance Program (EAP)

Amazon's free Employee Assistance Program provides confidential support, resources and referrals for various aspects of work and personal life. Help for parents whose children struggle with developmental disabilities is offered, as well as help finding child and elder care assistance. The company also provides access to financial counseling, estate planning and other services in the event of a life-threatening illness or death.

Employee Skill Development

Amazon's Career Choice program is an advanced education and career development offering. The program will pay up to $3,000 per year in tuition and associated fees for up to four years. The company also reimburses 95% of the cost of all required textbooks. Approved educational programs may not even have to be relevant to the associate's current position.

Periodic Performance Bonuses

Based on the achievement of high-level organizational goals, Amazon gives performance bonuses on a periodic basis. During 2020, all of us full-time employees received a mid-year bonus of $500, At the end of 2020, we all received an additional $300 bonus for solid performance during peak season. Part-time employees received a $150 bonus at the same time.

Paid Holidays

Amazon gives full-time employees six paid time off holidays for New Year's Day, Memorial Day, Independence Day, Labor Day, Thanksgiving Day and Christmas Day. This compares unfavorably with 8-10 paid holidays offered by the majority of U.S. employers.

Hourly employees earn time and a half if they work on any of the six Amazon holidays. This also compares unfavorably with the double time pay the majority of employers provide.

Free Safety Shoes

When I was first told that Amazon provides each fulfillment center employee with a $100 annual credit toward safety shoes, it triggered the skeptic in me. It did seem legit since the shoes came from Amazon's footwear subsidiary, Zappos. The story line was that while some Zappos work shoes were a little spendy, the $100 stipend would cover many of the shoes that were available with a little left over.

I could only laugh at the free shoe offer since I was certain the shoes we'd have to choose from would be the butt-ugly work shoes I've seen factory workers wear. I must admit I was wrong. I was impressed when I looked over the selection and prices. I ended up getting a nifty looking pair of Reebok tennis-shoe type of work shoes with steel toes. Awesome. Since it's an annual program, we get a new pair each year.

Amazon.com Employee Discount

Employees receive a 10% discount on Amazon products sold and shipped by Amazon.com. The discount does not apply to FBA products.

On-Site Medical Assistance

This is an area that involves a high degree of controversy so I must tread softly here. Amcare is Amazon's name for its on-site medical care operation. I point out the atmosphere of contention because a Google search will open a Pandora's Box of negative stories and opinions concerning Amcare. Personally, I've had nothing but positive results in seeking their medical assistance. Remember my wheelchair episode on my day three?

Other than my wheelchair ride, I only visited Amcare three times, and then only for minor ailments such as minor cuts, bruises and aching muscles. My research, however, uncovered many sad tales of more serious experiences supposedly had by less fortunate folks. There was even a sad story of an on-site death from alleged exhaustion in the early 1990s.

Similar to my research on other negative reports and opinions, I encountered lots of stuff written by disgruntled ex-employees and zealous news reporters. I read lots of stories about litigation against Amazon's Amcare but nothing I'd be willing to hang my hat on. Most of the stories have to be taken on faith. Since I have a very dim view of news media outlets, I generally put little faith in what they report unless it includes concrete proof.

In short, I'll hold back any serious commentary on Amcare and let you readers form your own opinions. I will make one key point, though. The naysayers' main contention is that Amcare creates a smokescreen giving the illusion that the company uses Amcare to keep people from seeking outside medical assistance. My experience refutes that claim. The Amcare folks who I saw when I had a problem were quick to advise me that if my condition continued, I should go to my own doctor.

Chapter 7

Coronavirus Contained

"If you don't like something, change
it. If you can't change it, change
your attitude."
-   Maya Angelou

The 2020 coronavirus epidemic turned pandemic caught Amazon and many other companies understaffed as they confronted out-of-season surges on the medical front. We all saw dramatically increased demand for anti-virus medications and new sanitation requirements to limit the virus's spread.

Amazon hired 175,000 temporary workers in the Spring of 2020, ultimately offering permanent employment to 125,000 of them. The company relaxed its work hour rules by allowing associates to take unlimited, unpaid leave as it implemented coronavirus safety measures. It also began widespread testing of the workforce. Testing was free and done on paid company time.

Employees who tested positive for the virus were given two weeks paid time off and more if needed. The company immediately put into place an internal employee tracing system. Any workers who were found to have come into close contact with co-workers who tested positive were also given paid time off for 10-14 days.

In spite of all the concerted efforts being made by Amazon to keep employees healthy and whole, media reporters dove into the weeds looking for negative stories. It did not take long for these super sleuths to isolate a few unhappy workers ready to strike out against big bad Amazon. Negative stories sprang up from questionable sources and outright troublemakers. This is not hyperbole on my part. I saw it in the local press with my own eyes.

In keeping with their pattern of never letting a good crisis go to waste, unscrupulous politicians seized the opportunity to spread the over-exaggerated claims and outright lies. In December of 2020, avowed communist Bernie Sanders tweeted, "Amazon workers are risking their lives to fill holiday orders and are denied paid sick leave." I'll have more comments on political lies in the next chapter. Even if I did not work at Amazon during the coronavirus pandemic, I'd know what an absurd falsification this was simply from my understanding of how Comrade Sanders has been telling bold-faced lies for years.

The problem is that many Americans, especially his fellow Democrats, believe him due to the notion that people would be sued for slandering people and organizations they don't like. Stephen Solomon, associate director of the Journalism Institute at NYU states, "Citizens attempting to sue public figures like politicians have to prove the slanderous claim was made on purpose or with reckless disregard for the truth. That's very hard to prove." So old Bernie sticks his head back in the sand and goes on his merry way.

Sanders is not the only one disparaging Amazon for its supposed indifference to keeping employees safe from the virus. Most anti-Amazon pundits jumped on the Bezos bashing bandwagon with high emotions and biting rhetoric. But, at the same time they had almost no factual information with the possible exception of a few tales of isolated incidents. Virtually none of these naysayers did any investigations to back up their claims of malfeasance. They totally ignore the facts I'm about to lay out for you.

All employees at Amazon's PDX9 facility were and still are advised immediately when any of their co-workers tests positive for the virus. The affected worker and any others found to have worked closely with them is given paid leave. After I received one such notice concerning a single individual, I was shocked to hear a local media outlet that had learned of the notification refer to the lone incident as an "outbreak" at the local Amazon warehouse. It was reported strictly for its panic-inducing value, meant to enhance the reputation of the errant reporter.

You don't have to take my word for this political and journalistic irresponsibility. A news article from Vox Media's *The Verge* entitled: *Amazon is giving paid sick leave to all employees diagnosed with coronavirus* shortly after the company took this action. The piece obviously went unnoticed by the Amazon antagonizers. *The Verge* piece outlined many of the precautions and preventive measures the company was taking to safeguard workers from the virus. "Amazon will give all employees diagnosed with the novel coronavirus as well as all those having been in close contact with them up to two weeks pay while in quarantine. That includes the company's part-time warehouse workers." Ever wonder why we never see any apologies or retractions from the misinformation perpetrators?

The news article went on to say "the company will establish a relief fund to help support its contractors and gig workers who are affected by coronavirus. The company's independent delivery service partners, Amazon Flex delivery drivers, and other seasonal employees who may experience financial hardship as a result of the ongoing coronavirus outbreak can apply for grants if diagnosed with the novel coronavirus or put into quarantine. Amazon's initial contribution to the fund, called the Amazon Relief Fund, will be $25 million. Grants from the Amazon Relief Fund will range from $400 to $5,000 per person."

Although Comrade Sanders and several other politicians were quick to prematurely chastise Amazon for its purported slowness in response to the coronavirus outbreak, FC management jumped into action. As soon as it became obvious that a 2-week shelter-in-place scenario was not going to suffice, actions were taken quickly to mitigate the spread of the virus among FC workers.

Facemasks were issued to everyone entering the warehouse facility and safety workers began immediately enforcing the wearing and proper fitting of the masks. Free virus testing was offered to all employees the minute test kits were made available by the government. All workers were strongly urged to get tested ASAP. Testing was scheduled in waves in a part of the warehouse set aside for that purpose and workers were administered tests during paid company time with statistical productivity tracking suspended.

Monitoring stations were set up at building entrances to take temperatures of everyone entering the building. Those who had temperatures above the prescribed threshold or displaying any symptoms of the virus were sent home with paid time off.

Safety personnel were hired to police the proper wearing of masks and adequate social distancing throughout the facility. To show how serious they were, these "coronavirus cops" wore special vests with "Keep your 6" emblazened on the back. I got the finger pointed at me more than once each day.

Disinfecting supplies were placed at almost every workstation and employees were strongly urged to use them regularly. Virus-spreading barriers in the form of mylar cubicles were constructed to make break rooms safer.

An almost constant flow of janitorial workers sanitized tables and other surfaces in breakrooms and work areas throughout the building.

Breakrooms were closed a few hours a day for disinfectant spraying and other sanitization activities.

Tables and chairs were removed from breakrooms to enforce social distancing, much to the chagrin of many workers looking for places to sit and relax during their breaks. I must admit I was a little pissed off when I could not find a place to sit while on my breaks, but I got over it. I often found a temporary seat on a small stack of pallets, upside down totes or work tables not in use. Of course, I was quickly chased from my perch by the green meanie safety police.

Immoral Profiteering?

While I'm always wary of shysters trying to take advantage of a suffering public during disastrous times, I was a bit bewildered by how quickly many politicians and the media severely criticized Amazon for profiting from the pandemic. If you step back and look at the big picture, I'm sure you'll be baffled yourself.

Did Amazon and Jeff Bezos profit during the pandemic? Of course they did. Did they plot a strategy to do so? As much as I distrust the motives of many giant conglomerates, my firm belief here is a definite no. Who in their right mind would craft such a conspicuously transparent scheme in the midst of a heavily publicized disaster? Is Jeff Bezos greedy? Probably so. But then what successful businessperson isn't. But, is he stupid enough to set himself and his company up for the devastating humiliation and public outcry surely to follow such an action? If you truly think he is crazy enough to put himself in such a dire predicament, you might want to have your own sanity checked.

In my opinion, it was simply a matter of being in the right place at the right time with a strategy that - with a humongous stroke of luck – just happened to provide an incredible solution to a very serious problem that popped up from out of nowhere. Or perhaps you think Bezos conspired with the Chinese to create and unleash the virus to put Amazon in the catbird seat. That would be the mother of all conspiracy theories.

The bottom line is this. Amazon's delivery service greatly assisted the millions of people forced to shelter in place. How many more people would have died had it not been for the company's ability to deliver such a vast variety of goods with record speed? They did not create that service for the purpose of profiting from a disaster nor did they raise prices to benefit from it. The business strategy was intended to earn substantial income by providing convenience to consumers. Should they be punished for stumbling into a fortuitous situation that gave them unanticipated rewards on a huge scale? I think not.

Chapter 8

Corrupt Politicians
Join the Fray

"If you tell a lie big enough and
keep repeating it, people will
eventually come to believe it."
- Joseph Goebbels

I've spoken throughout these pages on the subject of Amazon bashing. While disgruntled ex-employees and the media have been the haters maximus, a few opportunistic political figures couldn't resist the urge to pile on. As usual, these buffoons came without any meaningful facts.

Like the media, American politicians elevated Bezos bashing to somewhat of an absurd art form. It's a shame that so many naïve Americans have been duped by the misinformation and blatant lies being broadcast about both the company and its founder.

Nowhere in our society has outright lying become so commonplace and expected than in the political arena. It seems that politicians can tell whopper-size lies and are almost never held accountable. Libel and slander are crimes…except if you're a politician. The larger your reputation as a politician, the bigger your lies can be without ever being punished, financially or legally.

Donald Trump has been accused of lying by both media personalities and political opponents more than any president in recent memory. Trump's biggest downfall as a politician was his failure to refine his art of lying. Unlike most of his opponents, Trump's lies were not intended to be particularly hurtful to other individuals but rather to make his programs and accomplishments seem more impressive than they might otherwise be. In my opinion, these Amazon bashing politicians took great pleasure in doing as much harm as possible to Big Bad Amazon.

Bernie Sanders, Bold-faced Liar and Consummate Coward

In late 2020, Bernie Sanders, the self-proclaimed communist supporter, jumped on the Amazon-bashing bandwagon by lashing out on Twitter, "While Amazon is denying paid sick leave, hazard pay and personal protective equipment to 450,000 of its workers, Jeff Bezos has increased his wealth by over $70 billion." I was flabbergasted by the absurdity of this bold-faced lie perpetrated on the American public. Since this complete and utter fabrication was published while I was working in an Amazon warehouse, I can readily and honestly act as a knowledgeable fact-checker on this. With the exception of the single phrase about Bezos' wealth increase, every other word in the tweet is nothing but a slanderous misrepresentation…and even that phrase is simply an erroneous correlation.

During the 2020 Covid pandemic, Amazon responded to Sanders' ludicrous attack by stating the company had provided "more than 151 million masks" and "64 million ounces of hand sanitizer" to employees. In addition, the company was enforcing "mandatory temperature checks" and "social distancing." I saw this for a fact as I outlined in the earlier chapter on the pandemic precautions taken at Amazon facilities.

Along with Amazon executives' rebuttal to Sanders' disturbing lies, the company officially invited Comrade Sanders to tour a fulfillment center to "see for yourself" how it had made "the health & safety" of employees its "top concern." Sanders, ever the loud-mouthed coward, naturally refused the invitation to avoid being publicly humiliated.

While Sanders wealth is rather dismal in comparison to Jeff Bezos and Bill Gates, he owns three houses and is worth at least $2 million. How he amassed his small fortune without ever having done an honest day's work in his life is a story for another time, so I'll leave it at that.

Sanders defended his wealth by telling the *New York Times*, "I wrote a best-selling book. If you write a best-selling book, you can be a millionaire too." In digging a little deeper into this claim, we find Sanders dipped into his campaign fund to the tune of $445,000 for purchases of his own book. So, the reality is you don't have to simply write a book to become a millionaire, you have to have a campaign fund to make it a best-seller.

The purchase of thousands of copies of his own book was not the only way Sanders got around campaign finance laws for his own benefit. Since the 1970s, Senator Bernie Sanders, who has spent his entire career railing against the evils of the political establishment, has repeatedly directed campaign dollars to close relatives. As mayor of Burlington, Vermont, Sanders even directed substantial taxpayer funds to his wife.

Sanders put his wife on the Burlington city payroll and made a company of hers, Progressive Media Strategies, a top recipient of campaign cash. His congressional reelection campaigns paid one of his stepdaughters more than $50,000 over four years. A nonprofit his wife started, the Sanders Institute, paid her son, David Driscoll, a $100,000 salary.

On a related front, Joe Biden has a sister and son whose companies received large contracts from his last presidential campaign. About one-fifth of the $11.1 million raised by that campaign went to companies that employed close relatives.

The sad part of the story is that while such activity is surely unethical, it's totally legal.

On the civil side of the coin, if Jeff Bezos chooses to hire friends and family members to work at Amazon, he has to pay them out of his own pocket, not by appropriating taxpayer dollars.

AOC and the Great New York Debacle

Alongside Comrade Bernie Sanders sits another outspoken socialist who has crossed paths with Amazon. Alexandria Ocasio-Cortez, nicknamed AOC, made a colossal fool of herself on a national scale by taking a pathetic, losing stand against Amazon in a spectacular display of mammoth stupidity.

In the 2018 mid-term election, citizens of New York's 14th congressional district elected to the U.S. House of Representatives this 29-year-old waitress/bartender. AOC majored in international relations and economics at Boston University, graduating cum laude in 2011. Boston University is ranked #37 of American universities and #39 in the world by U.S. News & World Report, so it's a highly prestigious institution.

It boggles the imagination how a person can graduate with honors from a prestigious university earning a degree in economics no less, and yet seemingly have no knowledge of tax incentives, government subsidies and basic supply and demand principles. Yet AOC accomplished this feat.

Here's the short story of one of the most classic economic faux pax of the past few decades. AOC arrogantly claimed credit for torpedoing a deal New York's top politicians had struck with Amazon to build a second HQ facility in her own district. The deal would have brought "at least 25,000-40,000 good paying jobs and add nearly $30 billion to New York's coffers. AOC claimed the $2.8 billion in tax breaks Amazon would eventually receive was a waste of money that NY could use for other purposes. What she failed to understand is that a tax break is not real money that can be spent. It's simply a tax reduction on future income. That's taught in Economics 101. Duh!

"Won't you look at that: Amazon is coming to NYC anyway — *without* requiring the public to finance shady deals, helipad handouts for Jeff Bezos, & corporate giveaways," she wrote.

In a separate tweet, showing her sitting on a yellow bench, she added: "Me waiting on the haters to apologize after we were proven right on Amazon and saved the public billions." The smug look on her face shows she was totally oblivious to her amazing screw-up

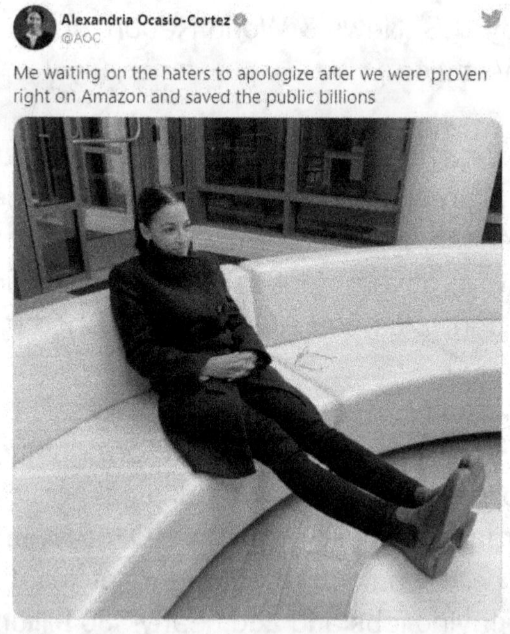

Amazon had promised to bring thousands of jobs to New York in exchange for up to $3 billion in tax breaks and financial incentives from the state and city governments.

"Anything is possible: today was the day a group of dedicated, everyday New Yorkers & their neighbors defeated Amazon's corporate greed, its worker exploitation, and the power of the richest man in the world," she wrote on Twitter after the deal collapsed.

Prior to running for Congress, AOC was a radical political activist and card-carrying member of the Democratic Socialists of America. Her highly vocal, controversial and charismatic personality and uncanny ability to get an abnormal amount of facetime on the national news put her in the limelight. She was able to position herself as the de facto figurehead of the Democrat Party. She used this power to transition the political platform of the Democrats to coincide with socialistic ideologies, stopping just short of full-blown communism.

So, putting politics aside, let's take a look at some of the ludicrous public proclamations Ocasio-Cortez has uttered during her first two years in office. Her erroneous and ill-informed statements have made her the laughing stock of many political pundits and a mockery of the House of Representatives. It's gotten to the point where her congressional colleagues cringe every time she steps up to a microphone.

Here is a sampling of some of her public rantings that make many people wonder if she was ever paying attention in school en route to graduating with honors.

- Showing her total lack of economics knowledge, she stated, "Unemployment Is Low Because Everyone Has Two Jobs"
- She mistakenly pointed out there are "Three Chambers of Congress," in her failed attempt to point out there are three branches of the U.S. government
- In a 2018 interview, Ocasio-Cortez claimed, "the American upper middle class doesn't exist anymore." At the same time, both CNN and US News and World Report estimated the upper middle class to include 28%-29% of the population. Income-wise, AOC together with all members of the House and Senate fall into the category. Is she saying she does not exist anymore?
- AOC's disdain for air-transportation security, protection from human and drug traffickers, anti-terrorist forces, disaster emergency services and biological-warfare defense is terribly dangerous. Yet she has continued to pontificate on these views in public.
- After reading a report about $21 trillion in Pentagon accounting errors over a period of 18 years in the past, AOC claimed "that money could be used to fund most of her proposed Medicare for All health care program." Anyone with a passing knowledge of economics has to know that accounting errors don't represent actual money that can be spent on something else.

All of the above statements come from a supposedly highly educated person. If AOC was a Republican instead of a Democrat, her all-too-frequent blunders picked up in sound bites would make her the darling of late-night talk show hosts. All the fodder for jokes she unwittingly produces seems to be non-stop. What does that say about the quality of education in America?

I feel sort of bad picking on poor little AOC because she continuously makes herself such an easy target. Keep in mind however that she's certainly not the only political figure to make people wonder whether she's ever attended any classes above the grade school level.

Given the debacle of almost single-handedly scuttling the proposed Amazon headquarters In Queens, AOC's own back yard, she remarkedly escaped any significant backlash she should have gotten for robbing thousands of her neighbors of promising job opportunities. Being a darling of the news media, most reporters and news anchors gave AOC a free pass on the issue. It was amazing to see her get re-elected after all the harm she did to her constituents.

Ilhan Omar, the Unconvicted (so far) Felon

Before launching into an expose on Ms. Omar, a little background on her is needed to fully comprehend the big picture vis a vis Amazon. Ilhan Abdullahi Omar is an American Muslim politician serving as the U.S. Representative for Minnesota's 5th congressional district in Minneapolis since 2019.

Born in Somalia, Ilhan and her family fled Somalia to escape war and spent four years in a refugee camp in Kenya. The family was granted asylum in the U.S. and Ilhan settled in a section of Minneapolis heavily populated by Somali immigrants.

Supported by her Somalian cohorts, Ilhan decided a career in politics was for her a quick and easy path to financial success. The fact that 'quick and easy' does not equate to 'legal and ethical' seems only to have brought out the worst in Ms. Omar. Instead of being grateful to the country that granted her asylum to escape hellhole conditions of her native country, she became a very vocal opponent of the American way of life and our free enterprise system.

As an active member of AOC's socialist squad. Omar was welcomed whole-heartedly by the Democrat party. She quickly became an outspoken activist for every socialist plank of the Democrat agenda including the Green New Deal, Medicare for All, open borders, elimination of ICE and other border security measures, Defund the Police, forgiveness of all student loan debt and free college for all. Not surprisingly, when asked where the money would come from to pay for all of these giveaway programs, Omar merely plays the bogus "tax the hell out of the rich" card.

It did not take long after being elected for Omar to join the ranks of the dirty politicians. This is not an isolated dig on the Democrats since there are dirty politicians on both sides of the aisle. In 2018, she was accused of campaign finance violations for using campaign funds to pay for personal travel, and divorce lawyer, among other goodies.

This opens up a Pandora's Box of dirty dealings aimed at skirting the law. The ever-manipulative Omar appears to have cleverly hidden details of her life that prompted accusations of immigration and tax law violations. Thus far, she has managed to dodge prosecution on these charges. Even the typically litigation-happy Internal Revenue Service is unlikely to pursue punitive measures.

A dark cloud of suspicion hangs over Omar's head when the subject of net worth comes up. While running for congress, Omar hired a male political consultant to work on her campaign. The two ended up having a romantic affair even though both were married at the time. They ended up getting divorced from their spouses over the tryst and Omar married her new lover. According to a *New York Post* article, Omar funneled about one-third of her campaign dollars to her husband as her consultant. According to his divorce papers, he was almost broke at the time of his divorce. After they were married, nearly one third of Omar's multi-million-dollar campaign fund went to her new husband. Technically, there is nothing illegal in this, but from a moral and ethical standpoint…well, as officeholders say, all is fair in war and politics.

…so, where was I in the conversation about Amazon?

Oh yes, back to Ilhan Omar vs. Amazon

In April of 2020, CNN published an article entitled "Fear and a firing inside an Amazon warehouse." It told the story of a 28-year-old Bashir Mohamed of Somali descent who had been working at Amazon's warehouse facility in Shakopee, Minnesota, a suburb of Minneapolis. Mohamed was employed as a "stower," a job he called "stressful."

Having worked as a stower myself for several months, I can attest to the fact that the only stress stowers feel is self-inflicted. It comes from a feeling of inadequacy of not being able to perform at a rate anywhere near the average of other stowers in the facility.

Mohamed's anti-Amazon activism started rather harmlessly as he merely began voicing concerns about the threat the China virus could pose to workers. His activist activities escalated as he began distributing paper petitions to his fellow workers and expressing concerns to management about what he called the impossibility of practicing social distancing in the warehouse.

Never having been to Shakopee, I did a little research to look into Mohamed's claim of "social distancing impossibility." Watching a few Youtube videos about the Shakopee facility, it looked like a carbon copy of the Portland facility, PDX9, where I worked. At PDX9, reasonable social distancing is not only possible, it seems to be pretty effective. Given the size of the workforce, incidents of covid-19 infections appear to be below average.

After having been given several warnings, Mohamed was fired for rules noncompliance. The company's official statement to CNN stated his termination was "a result of progressive disciplinary action for inappropriate language, behavior, and violating social distancing guidelines." Using PDX9 as a reference point and witnessing a number of confrontations between the Green Vests and social distancing violators, it is highly likely that Amazon's claims about the incidents involving Mohamed do hold water.

Ilhan Omar has become a sworn enemy of Amazon. She used the CNN article and a few other similar news clips in other cities to beef-up her anti-Amazon rhetoric. This is in spite of the fact that Amazon is pretty much the sole reason the Somalian community in Minnesota enjoys a great standard of living in comparison to the country they fled because of abusive conditions. Unlike Somalia, the U.S. is a free country and no one forces anyone to work for Amazon. It's each employee's personal choice.

Ilhan Omar and her buddies in the AOC 'Squad' blame Amazon for forcing "poverty like conditions" on the Shakopee community. This is in spite of the fact that the company pays $15/hour to starting employees, with increases taking that number to nearly $17/hour within a year. I saw my personal pay rate move automatically from $15 to $16.75 in seven months. The U.S. Department of Health and Human Services sets the federal poverty level at $26,200 for a family of four. That's equivalent to about $12.60 per hour for a full-time worker. By my calculation, Amazon is paying over 30% above the poverty level.

If Omar is so concerned about the welfare of Somalis in Minnesota, why does she not share some of her $2+ million net worth and her $250,000+ annual compensation package with her underprivileged comrades. Keeping with the personality traits of the spoiled brat she has become, we can be sure that will never happen.

* * *

These are only 3 examples of people who have no right to sit in judgement of a successful business person like Bezos or the successful enterprise he has built. Honest criticism is one thing, but lies coming from politicians is pure evil. They should just keep their mouths shut, feast quietly on their $250K+ compensation packages and wallow in their own parasite-like existence.

Throughout the book, I've pointed out lies and exaggerations spread my the media. Having said that, perhaps the number one source of mistruths is the political arena. Whenever a politician is extremely critical of a person or organization, you can assume their agenda is one of two possibilities with almost 99% certainty. They are either 1) trying to make themselves look good at the expense of others, or 2) attempting to destroy the reputation of someone they see as an enemy.

MEET THE AUTHOR

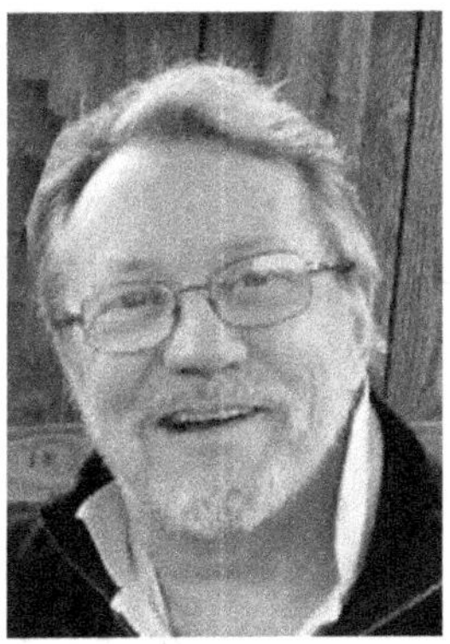

Emerging from a very modest upbringing in the Midwest with my eye on a more exciting lifestyle, I dropped out of high school and ran away from home to "do it my way" as Sinatra used to say. I was incredibly lucky that it worked for me, but I strongly recommend against such a strategy. I got my education later, but it was a tough road to travel.

Ever since that breakaway to freedom, I've had an unusual life experience to say the least. I've been broke a few times and a millionaire more than once, and I've enjoyed every minute of my life on the planet.

Totaling up the jobs I've held, the businesses I've founded and the organizations for which I've done consulting work, I've worked in 200+ companies across over 30 different industries. I would not trade that journey for anything in the world.

I've been a prolific writer, seminar presenter and public speaker internationally for over 30 years. I love sharing stories of my dazzling successes and the lessons I've learned from dismal failures. I'm fortunate the former outnumber the latter.

You can read more about my adventures and the lessons I learned along the way that led to a great deal of personal and business success in my book entitled: *Success Is Yours For The Taking…and Here's Where the Secrets Have Been Hiding.*

I'd love to hear your feedback about this book whether it be positive or negative.

Wishing you much success,

Dick Kuiper

You can email me at: dick@ghostwriterhelp.com